The Best Healthcare for Less

Save Money on Chronic Medical Conditions and Prescription Drugs

DAVID NGANELE, PH.D.

WILEY

John Wiley & Sons, Inc.

Published by John Wiley & Sons, Inc., Hoboken, New Jersey
Published simultaneously in Canada

Design and production by Navta Associates, Inc.

For general information about our other products and services, please contact our Customer Care Department within the United States at (800) 762-2974, outside the United States at (317) 572-3993 or fax (317) 572-4002.

Wiley also publishes its books in a variety of electronic formats. Some content that appears in print may not be available in electronic books. For more information about Wiley products, visit our web site at www.wiley.com.

Library of Congress Cataloging-in-Publication Data:

Nganele, David, date.
   The best healthcare for less : save money on chronic medical conditions
and prescription drugs / David Nganele.
      p. cm.
   Includes bibliographical references and index.
   ISBN 0-471-21849-9 (paper)
   1. Medical care, Cost of—United States. 2. Medicine, Popular. 3. Medicine, Preventive.
   [DNLM: 1. Health Care Costs. 2. Prescriptions, Drug—economics. 3. Health
Expenditures. QV 736 N576b 2003] I. Title: Save money on chronic medical conditions
and prescription drugs. II. Title.
   RA410.53 .N54 2003
   338.4'33621'0973—dc21
                                                                    2002153263

Printed in the United States of America

10 9 8 7 6 5 4 3 2 1

Contents

Appendixes

Foreword

The medical establishment has devoted a great deal of time to discussing healthcare disparities. There is a significant disparity between the insured, who have full comprehensive health coverage, and the underinsured, such as the elderly, who often have no pharmacy benefits. One could say the underinsured have enough insurance to die on but not enough insurance to live on. A lot of individuals with health insurance still have considerable out-of-pocket medical expenses for such things as copays and deductibles. As a society, we must find ways to close these healthcare gaps through political action and, more important, by educating the population at large on the best ways to negotiate the healthcare "maze."

The real issue now comes down to this question: Where do we look for answers to the problem of obtaining better healthcare? Fortunately, my friend and collaborator, David Nganele, Ph.D., has given us hope in his book *The Best Healthcare for Less*. This is a wonderful guide for any patient or healthcare provider who needs to survive the high cost of healthcare. The timing of this publication is such that those who work in the healthcare industry must take notice. A recent survey by the Kaiser Family Foundation found that physicians feel that health maintenance organizations and the managed care industry have decreased the quality of healthcare in the United States. The author is very astute in starting his book with a description of healthcare costs and where they come from. He uses a healthcare cost "pyramid" to illustrate the proportion of money spent at the different levels of healthcare. The healthcare cost pyramid shows how the present healthcare system often expends a small portion of its resources on prevention and huge amounts on what is at least partially preventable expensive hospital and nursing home care. Dr. Nganele then goes on to write about the most cost-effective care of all, preventative care.

One of the real strengths of the book lies in chapters 3, 4, and 5, which include a user-friendly flowchart for saving on prescription drugs. The author has a wealth of firsthand experience in the pharmaceutical industry, which makes his work in these chapters unparalleled. His use of case illustrations makes it easy for readers to apply the information to their own particular situations. But the greatest strength of these chapters may be that they provide information on cost savings for all consumers whether they are insured or not. The reader who desires more information will find a vast array of web sites, telephone numbers, and addresses to use as resources. The recent explosion of direct consumer advertising will cause the section on generic versus brand-name medication to be especially useful for the reader.

Because knowledge is power, the sections on the other areas of healthcare costs in chapters 6, 7, and 8 should give both patients and healthcare providers a good understanding of where one can effectively direct cost-cutting initiatives in healthcare without reducing services or quality. Importantly, the author also provides vital information on choosing a hospital, a physician, or a nursing home. In chapter 8, Dr. Nganele addresses employment and family issues, which are significantly affected by chronic illness. The literature shows that the great majority of the healthcare dollars spent on individuals are in the last years of life. We must all become familiar with the section on living wills and durable power of attorney, otherwise our elderly population will often receive procedures they don't need or will be denied services they should have access to, because of our ignorance about these issues.

In part four of his work, the author devotes entire chapters to individual diseases: Alzheimer's disease, arthritis, asthma, cancers, depression and anxiety, heart disease, diabetes, HIV and AIDs, and osteoporosis. The recent dramatic increase in the proportion of Americans over 65 years of age makes the chapter on Alzheimer's disease mandatory reading for everyone. Since I have a special interest in hypertension, I can highly recommend Dr. Nganele's chapter on heart disease, which gives a comprehensive yet concise explanation of how to work with your doctor to lower your blood pressure and decrease your risk of heart disease.

As a person who has seen the dramatic effect that mental illness can have on an entire family firsthand, I know that the chapter on depression and anxiety will be an invaluable resource for families who have previously known only frustration and despair. The high cost of managing HIV and AIDS now can easily exceed $20,000 per year. The author reveals that 20 percent of infected patients are not covered by health insurance. This book provides a solid overview of a very complex disease while offering a good reference list for those who want to obtain more information.

The appendixes found at the end of the book actually provide a state-specific list of pharmacy assistance programs and other health associations, which can be used to obtain assistance on prescription drugs and other resources. The tables are well organized and should bring clarity to an often-confusing process. The Internet addresses should also allow the consumer convenient online shopping. Lastly, it is important to note that the author does not neglect complementary and alternative medicine in this publication.

The U.S. healthcare system has been a leader in developing revolutionary and innovative technology, which often provides high-quality healthcare to a more elite few but does not address the needs of many others. One can only hope that the true value of primary prevention will be realized before our healthcare crisis becomes a healthcare catastrophe. This book is a positive step in helping to deal with the healthcare cost crisis.

Wallace Johnson, M.D.
Clinical Assistant Professor
Department of Medicine
University of Maryland School of Medicine

Acknowledgments

This has been an endeavor born out of passion—the passion to give unto others what I can to help them achieve a better quality of life. Passion sometimes has its price. For me that price has been one of diminished quality time with my family. I would like to dedicate this book to them and hope that somehow I can make up for that lost time.

My passion also could not have taken me to this point without the help and guidance of a lot of people. There are just too many for me to mention and I know I will commit the sin of omission. There are, however, certain individuals whom I have to acknowledge, just because.

To Charlotte Nganele, M.D., my best friend. I can't say anything that can truly capture what she means to me. For now, all I can say is thank you for being the friend you are.

To Katharine Sands, my book agent at the Sarah Jane Feymann Literary Agency. Katharine saw in me what I did not see in myself. She believed in me and never wavered in her enthusiasm and belief that I had something worthwhile to share with others. Yes, I was a pain sometimes, but she knew when to push and when to pull.

To Elizabeth Zack, my editor. It is truly amazing how she can give you directions to make your work so much better and yet still make you feel like you did it all by yourself. That is talent. I needed her guidance and patience, and she gave more than I could hope for.

To all my mentors—and you know who you are—please accept my gratitude.

Finally, I would like to acknowledge all who come across this book and find it helpful. That was my goal and if the information in here makes a difference in your life, my mission will be accomplished. Be well.

Introduction

A s you read chapter 1, you will see that all the numbers mentioned with regard to how much we spend on healthcare and what we spend it on measure only what we call *direct costs*—that is, the costs we incur when we receive services. There are lots of other costs, so-called *indirect costs,* that are not captured in these numbers. They include costs that result from lost productivity—when people are absent from work or from low productivity because they are sick—or when they die prematurely. There are also costs, called *intangible costs,* that we cannot put numbers on. These include pain and suffering and the emotional effect of being sick or dealing with a loved one or a relative who is sick.

Whether we have insurance or not, we pay more for healthcare out of our pockets than we think we do. The official numbers say that we pay for almost 16 percent of the cost of healthcare out of our pockets. That comes to about $20 billion a year. This number is actually very low because it reflects only what can be directly counted for by such things as drugs or healthcare services. Make no mistake: we pay much more out of our pockets for healthcare than we think. It doesn't matter whether you have health insurance. The money the government spends comes to the government in the form of taxes. The money that private insurance spends comes to it in the form of premiums. All of that is money that could have stayed in our pockets. When healthcare costs go up, the government increases taxes and insurance companies increase premiums to meet up with the costs. That means more money out of our pockets.

There are a lot of things you can do to manage the cost of health-care, especially when you are dealing with a chronic disease. You can take charge of your state of health and become the most important physician (and accountant!) in your healthcare. The more educated you become about your disease, what caused it, how it is controlled, and what it costs, both financially and emotionally, the better you will be at managing it and not letting it take over your life. In the end, you will be spending more of your money doing the things you enjoy doing instead of giving it to health professionals, as much as we love them and need them.

Good luck and be well.

PART ONE

Where We Are and Where We Should Be

CHAPTER 1

Healthcare Costs

Where They Come From and Who Pays for Them

The Cost of Healthcare

The cost of healthcare is now over a trillion dollars a year. The benefactors of this money transfer are:

Hospitals	$420 billion
Physician and clinical services	$289 billion
Home and nursing care	$133 billion
Drug Manufacturers	$130 billion

The rest goes to medical equipment and other services like dental care and research.

Take a look at the diagram on the next page. I call it the "the healthcare cost pyramid." Have you heard of the food pyramid? The food pyramid is a guide to help us achieve proper nutrition. The healthcare cost pyramid should serve as a guide to help us understand and, hopefully, control the cost of healthcare. A lot of money is being spent on healthcare; and the goal here is to show how we can spend wisely on healthcare and maybe even reduce the cost of healthcare by becoming educated consumers.

Explaining the Healthcare Cost Pyramid

Primary Prevention

At the top of the pyramid is primary prevention. Primary prevention is doing the things that prevent us from getting sick. This is achieved by living a healthy lifestyle, and it includes exercising, eating properly, and getting routine physical examinations. It also includes not doing the things that can get us sick, such as smoking, illegal drug use, and excess alcohol intake. As you can see from the diagram, this is the smallest section of the pyramid. *Primary prevention is the least costly thing we can do in terms of healthcare cost,* so we need to educate ourselves to do everything we can to stay in that section of the

Primary Prevention
(Exercise, Nutrition, Physicals)

Secondary Prevention
(Conventional, Complementary Therapy)

Institutional Care
(Hospitalization, Nursing Care)

The Healthcare Cost Pyramid

pyramid. While everybody should be living healthy lifestyles to avoid getting sick, there are certain individuals who are at high risk for certain diseases and they need to pay particular attention to what it takes to prevent getting sick.

It can't be repeated enough: *prevention is better than cure.* Prevention is less expensive, too. With primary prevention, you not only prevent diseases from starting, you might actually catch the beginning of a disease and do the things that prevent it from becoming a full-blown illness. Chapter 2 deals with primary prevention. The goal is to show how we can practice healthy living even when we think we don't have the time or we don't know what to do.

Secondary Prevention

As we move down the pyramid, we get into secondary prevention. Secondary prevention is doing the things that prevent an illness we have from becoming complicated. With primary prevention, we do the things that prevent us from getting sick. A lot of individuals can, for example, prevent getting diabetes by watching their weight through proper nutrition and exercise. Unfortunately, sometimes even with the best of efforts, we still get sick. When we do get sick, we need to understand all we can about the disease, what it is, how we got sick, what we need to do to treat it, and very important, what will happen if we do not manage it effectively. This is secondary prevention. Part 4 of this book considers secondary prevention in light of some of the major chronic diseases. I have focused on these chronic diseases because these are the ones that people have to live with for very long periods of time. So as you can expect, chronic diseases are the most costly to manage.

The most important physician in your life is you. The things you do every day to yourself will determine your state of health much more than anything any physician can ever do. Your physician can tell you all you need to know and do to stay healthy, but unless you do what's suggested, it will all amount to zero. And your negligence could cost you a bundle down the road.

So, what happens if your doctor tells you have high blood pressure, high cholesterol, or diabetes? You now fall to the middle of the pyramid. The goal here is to do everything you can in order not to fall to the *bottom* of the pyramid, that of institutional care. As you can see from the size of the box, institutional care is bigger than secondary prevention, meaning that it costs a lot more. We prevent falling to the bottom of the pyramid by strictly following the instructions from our doctors and other healthcare professionals. Whether we practice only conventional therapy, also known as Western medicine, or add on to that complementary or alternative medicine—in other words nonconventional medicine—the goal should be the same: to do what it takes to properly manage the disease.

Pharmaceuticals play an increasing role in helping us effectively manage diseases and keep us in the secondary prevention box. However, as the costs of medications go up, many individuals stop taking their medicines or take them inappropriately to save on the cost. While this might reduce expenses in the short run, eventually this poor disease management will result in the type of complications that will push an individual down to the bottom box of the pyramid. He or she might end up in a hospital or a nursing home, or worse, die prematurely. The key, therefore, is to find the means to get the needed medication and take it as prescribed. Because of the importance of drugs, I have devoted a whole section—part two—to prescription drugs, to show how any individual, regardless of insurance status or income level, can get medications at low or no cost.

Institutional Care

At the bottom of the pyramid is institutional care. This is where you now have to leave the comfort of your home to get taken care of, either in a hospital or a nursing home, because your condition now requires a greater level of management. This is healthcare cost at its most expensive state. Half of all direct spending on diseases goes toward institutional care. We pay that much for hospitals and other kinds of institutional care because they provide the intensive care needed to keep us alive—and for that, we truly owe them our lives. The point here is that they *are* expensive, and to the extent that we can do things to prevent going to an institution, to postpone going to one, to reduce the amount of time spent there, or to minimize what they have to do to us there, the less expensive the cost of healthcare will be.

Who Pays for the Cost of Healthcare?

The government pays for almost half of the cost of healthcare and private insurance pays for a third. Most of the rest comes out of our pockets. The programs that are available to help us with the cost include the different government and private insurance programs.

Government Programs

Government insurance comes mostly in the form of:
- Medicare
- Medicaid
- Child Health Insurance Program
- Coverage for the military

Medicare

Medicare was started in 1966 as a health insurance to assist the elderly. In 2000 it spent about $230 billion to take care of the medical needs of seniors and some disabled. The program is administered by the federal government. To have Medicare, you must meet the following requirements:
- You are age 65 or older.
- You receive Social Security or railroad retirement benefits.
- You or your spouse worked in a Medicare-covered employment for 10 years or more.

- You are a U.S. citizen or permanent resident, residing continuously in the United States for at least five years.
- If younger than age 65, you have a disability that makes you eligible for government aid, or have permanent kidney disease that requires dialysis or transplant.

There are two parts to Medicare: Part A and Part B. Part A, also called Hospital Insurance, covers the cost of hospitalizations, some nursing home cost, and some medical care at home, as well as hospice care. Most people get Part A automatically once they turn 65. There are no premiums to be paid for Part A. Part B, also called Medical Insurance, covers doctor's fees, outpatient hospital care, laboratory services, medical equipment, ambulance services, and other services that Part A does not cover. You do not get Part B automatically. You have to enroll in it, and pay a premium that is adjusted each year. For 2000, the premium was $50 a month and this amount is automatically deducted from your Social Security or retirement check.

Annual deductibles must be met for hospital stays ($800 in 2001), doctor's visits ($100 in 2001), as well as coinsurance for daily hospital stays and most other medical care. A lot of Medicare recipients buy supplemental insurance, also known as Medigap, to cover these costs.

There is a third part to Medicare called Medicare+Choice, sometimes called Part C. In Part C, a Medicare recipient who has both Parts A and B can choose to enroll in a Managed Care Plan that accepts Medicare. A lot of Medicare recipients enroll in this program because the managed care plans provide prescription drug coverage. Medicare itself does not provide prescription drug coverage, and that has caused a lot of heated debates because seniors are increasingly needing prescription drugs. In 2000, the average annual cost of a prescription for the top 50 drugs used by seniors was about $1,000. Since some seniors take up to 15 different medications, the cost of medications can become a great financial burden.

There are a number of programs, usually administered by various states, to assist Medicare recipients pay for some of their medical costs. These programs all have income eligibility; that is, you have to have an income below a certain level to qualify.

If you have questions about your eligibility to join Medicare or about the benefits, or to enroll, call the Social Security Administration at (800) 772-1213.

Medicaid

Medicaid was started in 1965 to help pay for healthcare for individuals with low incomes. It is jointly funded by the federal government and the states but is administered by each individual state. The federal government sets broad national guidelines but each state does the following:

- Establishes its own eligibility criteria
- Determines the type, amount, duration, and scope of services
- Sets the rate of payment for services
- Administers its own program

In general, for states to get federal funds, they must cover these individuals:

- Those with low incomes who meet the requirement for the State's Temporary Assistance for Needy Families (TANF) program, generally referred to as welfare
- People who are poor enough to be receiving supplemental security income (SSI)
- Children under age six and pregnant women whose family incomes are below 133 percent of the federal poverty guideline
- Recipients of adoption or foster care assistance
- Special protected groups, such as persons who lose SSI due to earnings from work or increased Social Security benefits, who may keep Medicaid for a period of time
- Certain Medicare beneficiaries who meet asset and income criteria

Because states have a lot of leeway in designing their programs, there is a lot of variation from state to state. Sometimes even within a state there may be different Medicaid programs.

Medicaid is more generous than Medicare in what it covers. Most states have added benefits to their programs that are not required by the federal government. This includes coverage for prescription drugs and payment for nursing home care.

To learn more about your eligibility for Medicaid and what services are covered in your state, call the state's health department. The phone numbers are listed in appendix A at the back of this book.

Child Health Insurance Program (CHIP)

This program was started in 1997 as a way to expand the State's Medicaid program to cover children who do not qualify for Medicaid. These are the criteria:

- Children under age 19.
- Family income below 200 percent of the federal poverty level ($34,100 for a family of four in 2001). Some states cover children in families with higher incomes.
- Must not be eligible for Medicaid coverage.
- Parents do not have to be U.S. citizens or even legal immigrants.

CHIP is very generous and usually covers:

- Well-child programs
- Immunizations
- Doctor's visits
- Laboratory and diagnostic tests
- Hospitalizations
- Prescription drugs
- Other medical services

States usually charge a small monthly premium that is based on income, sometimes as low as $4 per child per month. To learn more about your child's eligibility and how to enroll, call (877) KIDS NOW (877-543-7669) or your state's health office (see appendix A for the state's phone numbers).

Coverage for the Military

Present and past members of the armed forces have programs that provide them with health coverage and services. The most widely known is the Veteran Affairs (VA) Health System. There are 172 VA hospitals around the country. To be eligible for VA assistance:

- You must have enlisted in the armed forces before September 7, 1980.
- If enlisted after September 7, 1980, or entered active duty after October 16, 1981, you must have 24 continuous months of active duty service or have completed the full period of time for which you were called or ordered to active duty.

- You must have been discharged or released from active duty under conditions other than dishonorable.
- You must be recently discharged from the military for a disability determined incurred or aggravated in the line of duty.

Active duty and retired military individuals and their families can also use the various military hospitals around the country. Retirees and spouses and children of active duty, retired, and deceased members of the armed forces can be covered by an insurance program called the Civilian Health and Medical Program of the Uniformed Services (CHAMPUS). This program will pay for the use of nonmilitary medical services.

Private Insurance

Almost 100 percent of all large businesses (200-plus workers) and 60 percent of small businesses (three to nine workers) provide some type of health insurance for their employees. The health insurance coverage for employees usually moves in step with the economy. When the economy is soft, there is less coverage provided by businesses, especially small employers. The types of insurance coverage and the proportion of individuals with private coverage in these plans are as follows:

Preferred Provider Organizations (PPOs)	41%
Health Maintenance Organizations (HMOs)	29%
Point of Service (POS) plans	22%
Indemnity plans	8%

PPOs, HMOs, and POS are called managed care plans because the providers of care in these plans have agreed with the person paying the bills what services will be provided and how much each service will cost.

Preferred Provider Organizations (PPOs)

In PPOs, a network of physicians, hospitals, and service providers agree in advance on how much they will charge for their services. The fees for these services are usually lower than the providers would normally charge. Any member of that plan can see any doctor in that network or receive services from any institution that is part of the network. The beneficiary pays a percentage of the cost, and the insurance company pays the rest. If the patient uses a provider outside the network, he or she pays a higher amount for the services.

Health Maintenance Organizations (HMOs)

An HMO is like a PPO but more restrictive. In an HMO, you are given the names of primary care physicians (PCPs) from which you choose one as your "gatekeeper." Your PCP provides you with your basic medical care and is responsible for referring you to a specialist, also within the network, as he or she determines. When you visit your PCP or see a specialist when referred by your PCP, or use a network hospital, you pay a small copay and the insurance company pays the rest. If you see a physician other than your PCP without referral from your PCP, you will be responsible for the charges incurred. Some HMO plans, known as staff model HMOs, have their own healthcare facilities where they provide care rather than sending you to see doctors in private offices.

Point of Service (POS) Plans

POS plans are like HMOs except that if your PCP refers you to a specialist who is not in the network, the plan will still cover the charges. If you, the patient, however, decide to see a specialist or another physician who is not in the network, you will pay an amount that was already determined when you got the policy.

Indemnity Plans

These are known as conventional plans and are the oldest of the employer-sponsored health insurance plans. With indemnity coverage, you can see any physician you choose and receive any type of service you desire. The provider charges whatever amount it decides. You pay for the service until you reach your annual deductible, about $500 or $1,000. After you've met your deductible, the insurance company will then kick in and pay a percentage of your bills, usually 80 percent, of what it determines is the "usual and customary" fee. This means that the insurance company will look at the bill and decide how much it thinks the service should cost. The insurance company then pays 80 percent of that determined amount and you have to pay the rest. For example, if you get a bill for $500 and the insurance company determines that only $400 is allowable, the insurance company will pay 80 percent of $400, or $320, and you end up paying $180. Indemnity programs also have yearly maximum amounts that they will pay. Once they pay up to that amount, any other charges for that year that you incur will be your responsibility.

Challenges and Solutions for Small Businesses

In 2000, the average insurance premium for single (individual) coverage was $202 per month and $529 per month for family coverage. This represented an increase of more than 8 percent from 1999, far above the inflation rate of 3 percent. The trend of premium increases above inflation is expected to continue into the foreseeable future. The employer shoulders most of this increase since the share of the cost that workers contribute has not changed. Small businesses are particularly hit hard, because their premiums grew at an even higher rate (10.3 percent) compared to the 7.5 percent growth of larger companies. This puts a lot of small businesses in a bind: either absorb the premiums or cut out health benefits. Because most employers have come to realize that providing health benefits is good way to attract and keep valuable employees, they are reluctant to cut out health insurance benefits. There are a number of things, however, that a small business can do to manage the cost of healthcare:

- Set up Medical Savings Accounts (MSAs). These accounts are like Individual Retirement Accounts (IRAs). They allow the small business employer to provide insurance with high deductibles, which makes the policy less expensive. The workers then contribute money on a tax-free basis to accounts called MSAs to use to pay for these deductibles. The money accumulates with interest and if not spent, can be used toward retirement.
- Look into government programs for small businesses. Many state and local governments have set up special insurance programs to help small businesses buy health insurance at reduced costs. New York State, for example, has the Healthy New York program. Call your local chamber of commerce for information on these programs.
- Join an association. Many trade associations have created insurance plans for their members by pooling their resources. This

allows a small business to get the favorable treatment that large employers get. Explore the different trade groups related to your business and look into their insurance programs. If you find a good one, join and get the plan.

- Shop around. There are many services that act as independent health insurance brokers for small businesses. If you tell them what your needs are, they will present you with a number of choices from different providers and you get to choose which one best suits your needs. One of the largest of these is eHealthInsurance.com, which does most of its business through the Internet (www.ehealthinsurance.com).

- Encourage your employees to get involved in healthy living and effective disease management programs. In this book, we talk about what healthy living is and how to better manage various chronic diseases. Encourage your employees to learn more about what can be done to avoid getting sick, and if they get sick, how they can reduce the impact of that illness both medically and financially. You will benefit not only by reducing lost productivity due to absenteeism but may also reduce your insurance premiums by having a healthy workforce.

Many employees consider health insurance coverage so vital a benefit that they are sometimes reluctant to quit their jobs for fear of losing their health coverage. They end up, in essence, being hostages to jobs that they might not like and they become virtual prisoners of their employers. The government recognized this dilemma and passed two laws to help employees deal with this issue: the Consolidated Omnibus Budget Reconciliation Act (COBRA) of 1986, which allows an employee to continue health coverage for a period of time after he or she leaves a job, and the Health Insurance Portability and Accountability Act (HIPAA) of 1996, which governs preexisting medical conditions. These laws are discussed further in chapter 8.

Individuals in Search of Health Insurance

If you do not have health coverage, either through the government or through a private employer, you are left to find one for yourself. It is a daunting task, one that has left more than 40 million Americans with no health insurance coverage. If this is the case for you and you are seeking health insurance, you may be faced with a number of challenges:

- Insurance companies are reluctant to insure most people with preexisting medical conditions. If they do offer coverage, the premiums are extremely high.
- Many benefits such as maternity care, mental health, and prescription drugs are usually excluded.
- The application process can be long and very intrusive.

Some states have created laws to help control these practices. They include:

- Preventing insurance companies from eliminating coverage for preexisting medical conditions. These laws do not, however, force the insurance companies to accept an applicant, only that if the applicant is accepted then their preexisting condition must be covered. Insurance companies are then free not to accept an individual with a preexisting condition, or to accept one and charge much higher premiums.
- Creating high-risk pools to provide coverage for individuals who have been turned down because of their conditions. These policies are usually more expensive but do provide coverage that would otherwise not be available. An individual with AIDS, for example, would have a hard time getting regular insurance. A high-risk pool insurance would provide coverage for that individual.
- Creating laws that require health insurance companies to provide health insurance at premiums that are set on a market by market basis. This means that the state is broken up into different markets, and for each market the company creates a rate without regard to age, sex, or health status. Every individual in that market gets the same rate and benefits. For healthier individuals, these programs tend to be more expensive than regular plans.

If you are looking to buy health insurance, contact your state's department of insurance. Any company that sells health insurance in a state has to be licensed in that state and must comply with the insurance laws of that state regarding what it can and cannot do. Appendix A lists the phone numbers of the insurance departments of the different states.

CHAPTER 2

How Not to Get Sick

Primary Prevention

Prevention is better than cure—*and* less expensive than cure. So if we are going to discuss how to save on the cost of healthcare, we might as well start with the least expensive method: how to keep from getting sick in the first place. We can prevent a lot of diseases by living a healthy lifestyle.

The very essence of healthy living is simply to do the things that are good for our bodies and avoid the things that are bad for our bodies; it is that simple. However, since there are many things that are good for our bodies and many things that are not, let's list the main ones:

Things that are good for our bodies

- Regular exercise
- Proper nutrition
- Routine physical examination

Things that are bad for our bodies

- Smoking
- Excessive alcohol intake
- Illicit drug use
- Unprotected sex with multiple partners

Unfortunately, there are a number of reasons why many do not live healthy lifestyles or can't seem to do it on a continuous basis. The main excuses are:

1. It is not a priority.
2. They can't seem to find the time to do it.
3. It can be complicated and they just don't know what to do.
4. It is expensive.

The biggest stumbling block is that, for most of us, living a healthy lifestyle will cause us to change the way we live right now in some fashion. And change is hard. The good news is that we *can* change, and we do it all the time. If we understand how change happens, and then apply that to create a healthy lifestyle, we will achieve our goal.

Change begins as a result of a different mindset. Here are some of the reasons that people who successfully live healthy lifestyles use to keep themselves on the right track:

- I want to look good.
- I need to feel energized.
- I want to stay alive long enough to see my grandchildren.
- I hate going to the doctor or hospital.
- I don't like spending money on healthcare.
- My mom or dad or relative died from that disease and I don't want that to happen to me.
- I need to release stress.
- My doctor told me to.

Unfortunately, sometimes a reason is forced on us because something catastrophic happened. For example, it's often the case that when somebody has a heart attack, that person suddenly starts an exercise program, or when somebody has diabetes he or she starts thinking about diet and losing weight. *Don't wait. It will cost you a lot, both financially and emotionally.*

If you achieve the mindset that convinces you to live a healthy lifestyle, you would have taken care of excuses numbers 1 and 2 (not a priority and can't find time). You will make your healthy lifestyle a priority. Once you make anything a priority, you suddenly find that you can make time to do it.

Let's turn to excuses numbers 3 and 4, the complication and the cost. We will address these issues as we discuss the three basic things that you need to do to live a healthy lifestyle: regular exercise, proper nutrition, and routine physical examinations.

Regular Exercise

A lot of studies have shown the benefits of exercise on nearly every aspect of our lives. Exercise can lower blood pressure, control weight, and lower cholesterol. It can help us stop smoking, control stress, and sleep better. It can boost our immune system to help us fight diseases. It gives us strength and endurance. I can go on, and on, and on. In fact it is almost criminal, or it so it seems to our bodies, not to exercise. It would be hard to find anybody who doesn't think exercise is good for them. Fortunately, more and more people are adding exercise to their lifestyles. The bottom line: *Exercise is good for you, and is an essential part of a healthy lifestyle.*

Now let's consider some other aspects: exercise being complicated, and the money it takes to exercise.

Complications

We can discuss the different types of exercise: aerobic exercise and anaerobic exercise. We can talk about warm-ups, primary exercises, and cool-downs. We can talk about target heart rate. We can talk about target zones. We can talk about the training effect. Are these things important? Sure, and if you are an exercise physiologist, you'd better know them. Do you *need* to know them to exercise? Absolutely not. In fact, if you try to figure out all these things, you might give up because you might think it is too complicated.

So let's make things less complicated. Exercise simply means *doing an activity that increases the rate at which your body burns calories.* Calories are the bundles of energy that your body needs to do all the things it does to stay alive. We get calories from the foods we eat. If you think of exercise as increasing your body's activity level, then constantly doing the things that increase your activity level will give you the benefits of exercise.

Here are some of the activities you can do to burn calories:

Activity	Calories Expended per Hour
Rest and Light Activity	*50–200*
Lying down	80
Sitting	100

(continued)

(continued)

Activity	Calories Expended per Hour
Typing	110
Driving	120
Standing	140
Shining shoes	185
Moderate Activity	*200–350*
Bicycling (5.5 mph)	210
Walking (2.5 mph)	210
Cleaning car	220
Gardening	220
Laundry (outside drying)	220
Canoeing (2.5 mph)	230
Shopping	230
Golf (foursome)	250
Lawn-mowing (power mower)	250
Painting (house)	290
Fencing	300
Rowing a boat (2.5 mph)	300
Swimming (0.25 mph)	300
Calisthenics	300
Walking (3.25 mph)	300
Having sex	315
Badminton	350
Horseback riding (trotting)	350
Square dancing	350
Volleyball	350
Roller-skating	350
Stacking heavy objects (boxes, logs)	350
Vigorous Activity	*Over 350*
Baseball pitching	360
Ditch digging (hand shovel)	400
Ice-skating (10 mph)	400
Chopping or sawing wood	400

Activity	Calories Expended per Hour
Bowling (continuous)	400
Tennis	420
Dancing (square or folk dancing)	430
Lawn mowing (hand mower)	430
Shoveling snow	450
Hiking	460
Water-skiing	480
Hill climbing (100 feet per hour)	490
Aerobics (high-impact)	500
Basketball	500
Football	500
Skiing (10 mph)	600
Squash and handball	600
Dancing (rock and roll)	630
Bicycling (13 mph)	660
Rowing (machine)	720
Sculling (race)	840
Rowing (10 mph)	900

Source: Charles B. Inlander and the Staff of the People's Medical Society. *Men's Health and Wellness Encyclopedia: Everything a Man Needs to Know for Health and Well-Being* (New York: MacMillan, 1998).

Pick just one of these activities and do it and you will be exercising.

But having said that, follow these guidelines for a better and safer exercise program:

- If you have not exercised for quite some time and you decide to start a program, begin with low levels of activity and work your way up to vigorous levels of activity.
- If in the course of exercising you feel dizzy or out of breath or feel any type of pain, stop immediately and seek medical advice.
- Do not do any vigorous activity after a heavy meal. Wait at least two hours before engaging in a vigorous activity.
- If you are involved in a vigorous activity where you are sweating a lot, replace the loss with water.

The Cost of Exercise

A lot of people think that to exercise, they have to join a gym, buy fancy exercise equipment, have a personal trainer, or be involved in an exercise program. If you can afford all these things, great. But you do not need to spend a dime to have an exercise program. Got an old pair of sneakers? There are a lot of activities you can choose from the list on pages 19–21. If you need a program or someone to help you with your exercise, join an exercise group or start one in your neighborhood. You can also join less expensive clubs like the YMCA.

Proper Nutrition

The things we eat can have tremendous effects on our health. We can link some foods to causing diseases as well as link foods to helping us fight many diseases. Most people know that too much fat can block arteries, which can lead to a heart attack or a stroke. Most people know that being overweight can lead to diabetes. Most people know that certain processed foods can lead to cancers. Most people know of relatives, friends, or loved ones who developed an illness because of their lifestyle and the foods they eat. You might not have given much thought to proper nutrition. In fact, there are few people who give their bodies the right amount of all the nutrients. We are fortunate that our bodies, a lot of the time, can regulate themselves to get what they need and get rid of the things they do not need. We still, however, have to help our bodies because our bodies can only take this imbalance for so long before we start paying the price of poor nutrition.

To incorporate proper nutrition effectively into our lifestyle, we need to remember why we decided to live a healthy lifestyle and realize that to do that, proper nutrition should be a part of it. At its very core, proper nutrition is giving our bodies the right amounts of the essential ingredients our bodies need to live on. These are:

- Water
- Carbohydrates
- Proteins
- Fats
- Vitamins
- Minerals

How do we get these in the right proportion? The figure below shows the food pyramid developed by the U.S. Department of Agriculture.

In using this pyramid, we should eat *more* of the foods at the bottom of the pyramid and *less* of the foods at the top. Remember, it does not say "do *not* eat the foods at the top," just that we should eat *less* of them. This is important because our bodies need all the components mentioned above. Fats, for example, are needed by our bodies to maintain our brain function and other vital activities. If we totally eliminated fat in our diet, we would not function as well. Any attempt to deprive your body of any of these essential foods can have serious consequences. Another good example is when you deprive your body of carbohydrates (which is what happens when you go on an all-protein diet). Since carbohydrates are the main source of energy for the body, without them your body will start burning fat to release energy. This might sound like an answer to weight loss but, when your body breaks down fats to release energy, it produces substances that, in large enough quantities, can actually lead to comas and even death. So, to attain proper nutrition, resolve to eat more of the foods at the bottom of the food pyramid and less of the foods at the top.

A Guide to Daily Food Choices

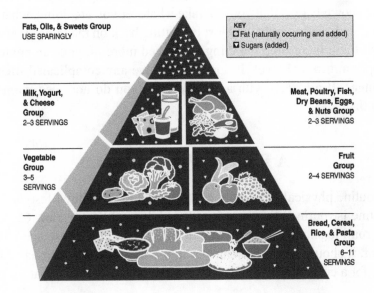

Fats, Oils, & Sweets Group
USE SPARINGLY

KEY
☐ Fat (naturally occurring and added)
☑ Sugars (added)

Milk, Yogurt, & Cheese Group
2–3 SERVINGS

Meat, Poultry, Fish, Dry Beans, Eggs, & Nuts Group
2–3 SERVINGS

Vegetable Group
3–5 SERVINGS

Fruit Group
2–4 SERVINGS

Bread, Cereal, Rice, & Pasta Group
6–11 SERVINGS

A Word about Vitamins and Minerals

Fruits and vegetables are very good sources of vitamins and minerals, but most times we are not sure if we are getting all the minerals and vitamins that are essential for our health. To make matters more difficult, our body does not store most vitamins and minerals: it takes what it needs at the time and gets rid of the rest. So, vitamins and minerals have to be replenished constantly. If you are not sure where to get the essential vitamins and minerals, and in what quantity, take supplements that give you 100 percent of the Recommended Dietary Allowance (RDA) of all the vitamins and minerals. They are inexpensive and you can at least be sure that you are getting what you need. The store brand is just as good as the name brands and costs much less. Also, choose multivitamins; don't buy multiple tablets. It is not essential to buy single formulations with very high doses of a particular vitamin or mineral. Most claims of what megadoses of a particular vitamin or mineral can do have not been substantiated. And for most of these formulations, your body will just use what it needs at the time and get rid of the excess.

The Cost of Proper Nutrition

Without even really considering it, we have addressed the issue of cost. The nutritional guideline specified does not involve any special recipes or the need to make any special efforts like joining a program. What I have shown here is that you can take whatever you are doing, what you are already eating right, and just by cutting back on the things you need less of and increasing the things you need more of, you can attain the proper nutritional level. It does not involve any complicated lifestyle changes. It all starts with a mindset, and you do not need money to buy that.

A Routine Physical Exam

A routine physical examination is essential to a healthy lifestyle. How routine is routine? For most healthy adults and those below 65 years, the routine should be every one to three years. For those age 65 and older, it should be every year. If you are in a category that has a high risk for a certain disease or you have a medical condition that needs to be followed up closely, your doctor will determine how often you need to come in for a checkup.

A routine physical is important because a lot of diseases are "silent killers." This means that for the most part, at least at the beginning stages of the disease, you have no symptoms and you do not feel any pain. By the time you start feeling symptoms, it might be too late or the disease might have progressed to the point where it is now more complicated and hence more costly to manage. Such diseases like high blood pressure, high cholesterol, diabetes, and even AIDS can go unnoticed for years in our bodies. For a lot of individuals, the first time they know that they have a disease is when something catastrophic happens and they need to see a doctor immediately. So as part of maintaining your body health, don't wait until the next physical if you are experiencing symptoms or feelings that you know are not part of how you normally feel. This is a way your body tells you that there is something wrong. Besides, it's been shown that individuals who have an established relationship with a particular doctor or medical establishment have a better health status than individuals who have not established such a relationship. This is because your medical history is better known, and a plan can be established for when you need to get evaluated based on your history.

Cost Issues Related to Routine Physical Exams

Physical exams are usually not expensive and a lot of insurance companies actually waive the copays to encourage members to have one. Many organizations and institutions also provide free screenings and educational programs.

If You Have Insurance

If you have insurance, make a point of scheduling a routine exam with your doctor. You are most likely not going to pay more than a few pennies for it. Check with your plan about its coverage policy regarding physical checkups.

If You Don't Have Insurance

Take advantage of programs that are held in the community by various organizations. Many churches, for example, hold health fairs that provide screenings for conditions such as high blood pressure, diabetes, and high cholesterol. Health fairs are also held in schools, malls, and senior centers. A lot of health organizations hold programs in the community as well. If there is a particular disease for which you are at high risk—for example, if there is a history of diabetes or cancer in your family—you might want to contact the various organizations or advocacy groups for that disease. These groups can provide not just education regarding the disease, but also information on where to get assistance with costs. Part four of this book provides the phone numbers of various advocacy groups for the various chronic diseases discussed.

Another way to get a free physical exam is to take part in a clinical study. Just be sure you would like to be part of the study, as opposed to just getting a free physical exam. Many teaching hospitals will provide free physicals as part of either a clinical study or for teaching purposes.

If you can't find free physicals, it still pays to go to a doctor and get an exam, especially if you are in a high-risk group or you believe that there is something wrong. The cost of taking a physical exam is much less than the cost of not detecting a disease or waiting to treat it when it becomes more complicated. It pays to shop around. When you go for a physical, ask about the tests that are relevant to your particular situation and get only those. Some clinics and hospitals will examine you and charge you based on your income. They can also arrange payment plans to meet your needs.

You should now be in the frame of mind to work toward disease prevention and be on the road to saving money on healthcare.

PART TWO

Prescription Drugs

CHAPTER 3

Prescription Drugs and Healthcare Cost

D rugs today have not only caused us to live longer but they have also improved the quality of our lives. A lot of illnesses can be managed effectively with medications, reducing the need for hospitalization or nursing care. Thus, medications are cost-effective in managing our diseases. Newer and better drugs are being developed each year.

Many people, however, struggle with how to afford prescription drugs. The elderly, those 65 years old and older, are especially hit hard. This group, which is expected to double by the year 2030, uses about 35 percent of all prescription drugs.

The classes of people most affected by the high cost of prescription drugs are:

- People who have no health coverage.
- People who have health insurance but their policy does not provide prescription drug coverage. This applies to seniors on regular Medicare since Medicare does not provide prescription drug coverage.
- People who have insurance coverage but are given prescriptions that are not covered by their plan. This applies to individuals with managed care coverage who have been given a prescription for a drug that is not covered by the plan.
- Individuals with prescription coverage, especially those on multiple medications, who face increases in their share of the cost of the drugs.

The debate over the cost of prescriptions is often complex and emotional. Drug companies are in the business of producing drugs for a profit, and they have done a great job in producing newer medications that work better or safer than older medications. It costs a lot of money, to the tune of over $500 million, to get a product to the market effectively.

The debate has always centered on how much these drugs should cost. Drug companies need to get back the money spent in developing a new drug, but more importantly, they need the profits to be able to have enough resources to fund the research to produce the *next* generation of drugs. Most of the new drugs used around the world are developed in the United States. This is because the U.S. market is the only market that allows drug companies to price their products using market forces as opposed to the government imposing price controls. This does not mean that drug companies can charge whatever they want. Market forces prevent them from doing so. Competition within the industry, either from other brands or from generics, when available, helps to ensure that drugs are not priced as much as the manufacturer might like.

Another market force in play is demand for the drug. Newer medications usually are safer or work better than older medications. The drug company might have to spend a huge amount of money educating the public about the drug, in the form of advertisements and consumer brochures, to create a demand for the newer medication. With greater demand, the company can charge a bit more, just as the manufacturer of any product might be inclined to do.

As stated in chapter 1, prescription drugs play a major role in secondary prevention. With most chronic diseases, the proper use of prescription drugs can effectively prevent or delay the need for institutional care, thereby saving a lot of money. Many individuals, however, do not take their medicine as prescribed or don't take it at all. One of the biggest reasons for this is that these individuals cannot afford the medication. Chapters 4 and 5 address this problem. Whether you have insurance or not, whether you are rich or poor, you can always find a program that will allow you to have access to any medication, either for free or at markedly reduced prices. Using the programs described here, cost should not serve as an excuse, especially when you are dealing with the most important aspect of your life: your health.

The chart on page 32 provides an eight-step process that you can use to determine which program, or programs, can best meet your needs. (Note that this is only a summary of the programs. Chapters 4 and 5 go into details and give you step-by-step guides on how to use them.)

Understanding the Steps

Step 1. The first step when you are given a prescription is to figure out if you have insurance that covers that particular medication. If the answer is yes, use mail order and samples to realize savings even when you have drug coverage. If you do not have insurance or your insurance will not pay for the prescription, move on to step 2.

Step 2. Is it an acute condition where samples can be sufficient? If yes, ask your doctor for assistance in obtaining samples. If it is a chronic condition, samples might not be sufficient and you need to move on.

Step 3. The next "no cost" alternative to samples is direct assistance from drug companies. Look up the manufacturer and call the company to see if you qualify for its assistance program. If you are not sure how to go about this process, use one of the services that assist patients with these programs. Some drug companies now offer their medications at a discount for seniors on Medicare who have no prescription drug coverage and don't qualify for the free drug program.

What if you don't qualify for the drug company's program or the company doesn't have an assistance program? Go to step 4.

Step 4. Check to see if your state has a prescription assistance program. Do you qualify for the program? If yes, apply and make use of it. Remember that it takes time to get enrolled in these programs. While you wait, you may have to use other means to get the drug, such as samples or paying for it at the local pharmacy.

What if you do not qualify for the state's program or your state doesn't have a drug assistance program? Move on.

Step 5. Ask if there is a generic version of the drug. If there is, request the generic drug through your doctor. If no generics are available, go to the next step.

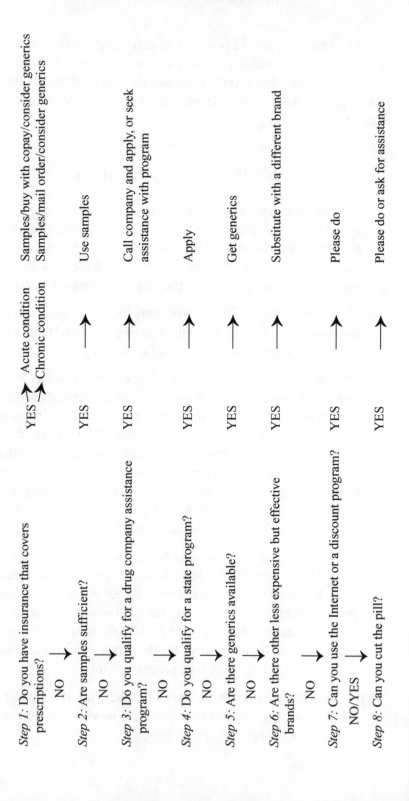

Eight Steps to Saving Money on Prescription Drugs

Step 1: Do you have insurance that covers prescriptions?
→ YES → Acute condition → Samples/buy with copay/consider generics
→ YES → Chronic condition → Samples/mail order/consider generics
NO →

Step 2: Are samples sufficient?
→ YES → Use samples
NO →

Step 3: Do you qualify for a drug company assistance program?
→ YES → Call company and apply, or seek assistance with program
NO →

Step 4: Do you qualify for a state program?
→ YES → Apply
NO →

Step 5: Are there generics available?
→ YES → Get generics
NO →

Step 6: Are there other less expensive but effective brands?
→ YES → Substitute with a different brand
NO →

Step 7: Can you use the Internet or a discount program?
→ YES → Please do
NO/YES →

Step 8: Can you cut the pill?
→ YES → Please do or ask for assistance

Step 6. Inquire if there is a less expensive but equally effective brand name drug. If so, ask for that substitute.

What if there are no generics and no other brand is as effective, and you have to buy that particular brand? You still have the following alternatives (see steps 7 and 8).

Step 7. There are ways to buy drugs at discounts to the retail price that you would normally pay at the local pharmacy. This includes buying the drug through the Internet or using a discount pharmacy program, where you can save as much as 50 percent over retail. Also, see if the manufacturer of the drug has a discount program. To realize even more savings, move on to the last step.

Step 8. Did you consider pill cutting? Be sure to check with your doctor or pharmacist to ensure that it is safe to do this for the drug in question. If you can use the pill-cutting technique with your medication, you can realize even more savings.

These steps will allow you to obtain the medicine at the least expensive cost. The next two chapters will describe these programs in detail, and provide a step-by-step guide on how to use each one.

CHAPTER 4

Saving on Prescription Drugs When You Have Drug Coverage

If you have insurance that covers prescription drugs then you don't have to worry about medication cost, right? Well, maybe or maybe not. Most probably, when you get a prescription from your doctor, you take it to your local pharmacy, and if you have managed care insurance, you pay a copay—your share of the cost. The pharmacy then deals with the insurance company to get paid the other part of the medication cost. Most individuals have health coverage through managed care plans, and these plans provide prescription drug coverage with copays. The copays are usually fixed amounts, between $10 and $30, depending on what the plan designates in your contract. Usually the amount is fixed for a year, and that is how much you pay, regardless of the actual cost of the medication. So, if the medication costs $100 and your copay is $10, you pay $10. If your doctor prescribes another medication that costs $200, you still pay only $10. Your insurance pays the difference to the pharmacy. Many managed care plans are now developing different copays for members based on the plan's cost for the medication. So, for example, a member might be charged a copay of $10 for the generic version of a drug but will have to pay a copay of $30 for the brand name.

There is a catch to the copay system, however. For you to pay only the copay, your doctor must prescribe a medication that appears on what is called a formulary, which is the list of medications that the insurance company has decided it will pay for. If your doctor decides that the medication that is the most appropriate for you is not on the formulary, he or she has to call the insurance company to justify its use. If the insurance company is not satisfied with the explanation, you will have to pay the full price of the medication.

If you have indemnity insurance that covers prescriptions, you pay for the medication and then submit a claim form to the insurance company to get reimbursed for all or part of the medication cost.

In all of the above cases, the out-of-pocket costs are usually small and most people who need medications for an acute condition can easily manage the cost. It starts to be a bit more complicated and expensive, however, when an individual has several chronic conditions and/or is on several medications. Even when you obtain your medications with copays alone, if you have several chronic conditions such as high blood pressure, high cholesterol, and diabetes, and are on several maintenance drugs, these copays can add up pretty fast.

The first step in managing the cost of prescriptions is to determine if the disease is an acute condition or a chronic condition. Acute conditions are illnesses that usually come on suddenly and whose treatments require relatively short periods of time, from a one-time therapy to a month or two of medications. Examples of acute conditions are pain after you see a dentist, an infection such as a strep throat or an ear infection, or a cold. Managing these conditions is not as expensive because once the treatment regiment is completed, the disease is usually cured.

Chronic conditions, on the other hand, usually develop gradually and when diagnosed, have to be treated for longer periods. Chronic conditions like diabetes and high blood pressure have to be treated for longer periods of time, even for life. It is important to realize that with these conditions, you have to continue treating the disease even when you do not feel any symptoms. Many of these diseases have to be "managed" because we do not yet have cures for them. When patients fail to follow treatment directions like taking their medicine every day, the disease can become more complicated and more difficult to manage. The result is an even greater expenditure on healthcare.

There are two strategies for managing the cost of prescriptions when you have coverage: mail order and samples.

Mail Order

Mail order is one of the least used and yet most effective means for saving money for those on chronic medications who have insurance coverage. To demonstrate: If you are a member of an HMO and you are given a prescription, you usually have it filled at a local pharmacy that accepts that insurance. If you are on chronic medication, such as a high blood pressure medication, you will be given a 30-day supply and be told to refill it as you approach the end of the 30-day supply period. You pay a copay every 30 days.

With mail order, you can request that your doctor give you a prescription for up to 90 days. You then send the prescription, along with your usual copay, to the pharmacy mail house that the insurance company has hired to manage its prescription drug program. The medication is sent to you by mail. The copay is about the same as the 30-day-supply copay you would incur at the local pharmacy. That means you are *getting a 90-day supply for the same price as the 30-day supply.* If your copay were, say, $25 a prescription, you would have paid $75 to have filled it three times at the local pharmacy. By using the mail order, you might pay only $25 dollars for a 90-day supply, saving $50. Over time, or if you are on several medications, this can amount to substantial savings.

Mail order pharmacies are able to offer such reduced costs because they deal in large quantities. They do not have to operate individual stores or pay a huge staff.

Pharmacy benefit managers (PBMs) operate most mail order companies. PBMs are companies hired by health insurance companies to help them manage the drug side of their business. Some of the largest PBMs are Diversified Pharmaceutical Services (DPSs), Express Scripts/ValueRx, and Merck-Medco.

The advantages to using mail order to obtain prescription drugs include:

- Mail order is cheaper than going to your local pharmacy.
- You maintain your privacy and get home delivery.
- Mail order operations have become very sophisticated with computers that check and recheck prescriptions to ensure that there are no prescription errors.
- If you have been with your insurance company for any length of time, the PBM will have a history of your medication. The mail

order company can therefore detect if you are being given a medication that might cause a drug interaction with another medication you are on. This ability to catch a potential drug interaction might not be available at your local pharmacy if you have used different pharmacies to fill different prescriptions.

- Mail order companies are usually designed to handle chronic medication schedules. This allows them to call you and remind you when you have to refill your prescription.
- Most PBMs have web sites where you can view your medication history, order medications, and review procedures.

Issues regarding mail order operations include:

- It takes time. Do not use mail order for acute situations, such as when you need an antibiotic for an infection. Mail order operations may take up to two weeks or longer to process and deliver your medicine.
- When you order drugs by mail, be sure to make arrangements for proper delivery and handling when the drug arrives. This means that you have to be aware of extremes in temperature if the medication is to be left in a mailbox. If the temperature gets too hot or too cold and the medications are exposed to these extremes for long periods, they might get damaged.
- Also be sure the medicines are not delivered and left in an area where children can access them and mistakenly ingest them.
- Using a mail order pharmacy also takes away the personal touch you might have with your local pharmacy. You may be the type of person who finds this personal touch valuable and decide it is worth the extra money to have the reassurance your local pharmacist can bring. However, all mail order companies have customer service numbers that let you speak to a licensed pharmacist.

To order prescriptions by mail:

1. Call your insurance company and obtain the phone number of the company that manages its mail order services or inquire about the mail order services of discount pharmacy programs or Internet pharmacies.
2. Call the mail order company to request the procedure for using the mail order system.

3. Request from your doctor the maximum number of days of prescription allowed by your plan.
4. Request the maximum number of refills allowed.
5. Submit your prescription, with your copay, either by phone, fax, or mail.
6. You should receive your medicine within two weeks.

Samples

Samples are free medications provided by drug companies to physicians, to give to their patients. Samples are very useful, especially in acute disease states when the patient needs medication immediately and can't wait to get a prescription filled in a pharmacy. Pharmaceutical companies provide samples to physicians to start new patients on the drug to determine if the drug might work for the patient before committing them on the drug long-term. Samples also create brand awareness and build product loyalty.

Samples can save you a lot of money. Doctors, by law, cannot charge for samples. In many acute conditions, such as a routine strep throat infection or acute pain, the physician might have enough samples to cover the whole course of treatment. If your doctor, therefore, gives you a prescription and you can't afford it, ask the doctor if he or she has free samples. Your doctor might have enough for the whole treatment or might have some to get you started and then you can fill the rest at the pharmacy, hence saving you money.

While samples are not ideal for chronic conditions, they nonetheless can be useful in chronic conditions as well. Your doctor might have "stock" bottles of medications. Usually samples are packaged to contain just a few pills to get you started on the drug. That's why samples are also referred to as starters. For chronic conditions, some drug companies provide physicians with containers that have up to a month's supply. Physicians have been known to sustain patients who cannot afford to buy medications for months on these stock bottles.

There are many benefits to using samples:

- Samples are free. They have been used effectively by physicians to assist a lot of individuals who could not afford the price of the medication.

- Samples result in high compliance. Many individuals do not fill the prescriptions their doctors give them. With samples, however, the patient is getting the drug directly and has a higher chance of treating the condition.
- Samples help the doctor know if a particular medicine will work for a patient and if there are side effects that would make it wiser to switch to a different drug. Medicines do not all have the same effect on all patients, and other medications could be available for the same condition. By giving a patient samples for a short period of time, a doctor can determine if that patient should stay on that drug or try a different one.
- Samples help physicians become more familiar with new drugs. When a new drug comes out, the drug company promotes it heavily and gives out lots of samples. While the patients benefit from this new therapy, the physician has the chance to evaluate for himself or herself how the drug really works. It also allows the doctor to know if there are special patient types that the drug works better in, any special conditions or circumstances to keep an eye out for, and any dosage adjustments that need to be made.

Certain issues must be kept in mind as far as samples are concerned:

- Your doctor might fail to catch an important drug interaction. In a regular prescribing sequence, a patient receives a prescription from a doctor and uses a pharmacy to get the medication. With samples, the patient gets the medication directly from the doctor. In nearly every case, this works just fine. Pharmacists, however, play a role in catching medication errors and in checking for drug interactions. If a pharmacy is not involved, it makes even more sense to ensure that your doctor is aware of what medications you are taking, including herbal medicines. If you have any questions as to what you received, go back and ask your doctor or consult with your pharmacist. Another circumstance where a pharmacy can be of help is in the case where a medicine has been recalled because of safety or other concerns. If the pharmacy has a record that you are on the drug, at least another person besides your doctor can notify you.
- Samples might not be properly managed. Federal law, state law, and private regulatory bodies require the proper handling, stor-

ing, and accounting of samples. There have been circumstances, however, where samples were not being properly handled or patients were given medications that were no longer useful. Although this is rare, ask your doctor if you have any doubts. Also check the expiration date on the package you are given to ensure that the medication is still good. A word of caution, though, about expiration dates: expiration dates do not always determine when a drug stops working. So your doctor might give you a drug that has recently gone past its expiration day. Bring the issue up with your doctor. If the expiration day was not that long ago, your doctor may say it is fine to use.

- Be sure you are getting your sample from a person who is authorized to give you a prescription. While office staff members help the physician or prescribing personnel hand out medication, they can only do so with written orders from the prescriber. Be sure you are getting samples as a result of your doctor's orders.

- Samples could cost you more money in the long run, because physicians give out samples of what they have and samples in physicians' offices tend to be of new products that are usually more expensive than older drugs. So, if you have a chronic condition and you were started on an expensive product, although it was free at the beginning, staying on it might become costly in the long run. If you are given samples of an expensive medication, be sure the samples are enough to cover you for the course of the treatment. If not, ask your doctor if a lower cost drug is available, which, although you might have to pay for it, ensures that over time you come out ahead financially.

About Drug Vouchers

Physicians normally get samples through sales representatives from pharmaceutical companies based on their specialty and prescribing habit. The practice location also determines what type of samples they receive. For example, office-based physicians get more pills and less of the types of products that are used in hospital settings such as drugs given intravenously.

A growing number of hospitals and other health institutions are now banning the use of samples, however. The reasons range from the difficulty of maintaining proper handling and management of the samples as required by regulatory bodies to the effect of drug samples on cost. An alternative to samples is the use of *drug vouchers*. With drug vouchers, patients receive a coupon for the drug, which they take to the pharmacy to receive the medication for free. The drug company reimburses the pharmacy for the cost of the drug.

Resources

For a complete listing of mail order companies, visit the web at www.managedcareregister.com. To learn more about samples, call the National Association of Boards of Pharmacy at (888) 481-9474, or visit their web site at www.nabp.net.

CHAPTER 5

Prescription Drugs at No Cost or Low Cost

With or Without Insurance

In this chapter, we discuss the various programs that would allow any individual, regardless of insurance status, to save on prescription drugs. We will first discuss the programs that drug companies have to give free medications to those who qualify. We will then explore programs that can significantly increase savings on the purchase of medications.

There are three situations where an individual has to pay for prescriptions:

1. When they have no health insurance
2. When they have health insurance but that insurance does not cover prescription drugs, as is the case with Medicare
3. When they have insurance that covers prescription drugs but their physician prescribes a medication that is not on the formulary of the plan and the patient is refused coverage for that particular medication

Prescription Drugs at No Cost

Two programs can provide free medications for individuals: samples (see chapter 4 for details) and drug company patient assistance programs.

Drug Company Patient Assistance Programs

Nearly every major pharmaceutical company has a program to help those who cannot afford their medications. Each company has a number of criteria that have to be met for an individual to obtain free medication. Basically, there are two main criteria: insurance coverage and income.

Insurance Coverage

To qualify for assistance, you must not have any other health plan, either private or public, that covers prescription drugs. This means that even if you have health insurance, such as Medicare, as long as that insurance does not cover prescription drugs, you might still be eligible. Also, there should not be any state program that can cover you for that condition. So check with your state to see if you qualify. Just remember that even if your state has an assistance program, a special medical situation might allow you to qualify for assistance from a drug company.

Income

Usually, the patient must not earn above a certain income level to qualify for these programs. Sometimes the particular company states what that amount is, but in many cases there are no exact amounts that a company considers a cut-off point. These companies base their decisions on a "hardship criterion." In other words, you need to demonstrate that the cost of the medication represents a hardship to you because of your financial situation. You might earn up to $50,000 a year and still be eligible if your medications represent a significant portion of your expenses. Even a temporary hardship, such as a job loss or a divorce, can still allow you to qualify.

After you demonstrate that you have met its criteria, the drug company will send the medication to your doctor, who then gives it to you. Sometimes you can pick up the drug at your local pharmacy.

This program should be used for chronic conditions because the review process takes about two weeks or even longer, and obviously you can't wait two weeks to treat a strep throat.

The companies usually supply from one to three months' quantity of the drug. At the end of that period, the patient must recertify that they still meet the eligibility criteria to continue receiving the free medications.

Issues Related to Drug Assistance Programs

While assistance from drug companies is one of the largest sources of support available, there are drawbacks to using these programs.

- The process can be slow. It takes between two and six weeks for the patient to get the drug. These programs, therefore, are not a viable source of support for acute conditions where you need the product immediately. For chronic conditions, however, it is usually worth the wait.
- Each drug company has its own set of criteria for eligibility and its own rules for obtaining their medications. If you need two medications, the fact that you qualify for the program with one company does not guarantee that you will qualify for the program with another company. Dealing with a different drug company for a different drug means starting the whole process all over again.
- The biggest drawback to these programs is the amount of paperwork and number of procedures that have to be endured to actually end up getting the drug. Many companies have tried to simplify the procedures but a lot of them still require a fair amount of paperwork. Many people get frustrated and sometimes give up.

To deal with all the paperwork and aggravation, a number of companies are available to assist individuals with the patient assistance programs from drug companies. Two such companies are the Indigent Patient Services and the Medicine Program.

Indigent Patient Services

You can contact Indigent Patient Services at the following numbers and at their web site. (Note: All numbers and web addresses are current at the time of this writing, but are subject to change.)

Phone: (727) 821-7333
Fax: (727) 898-0004
www.gihs.com/ips

To use Indigent Patient Services, follow these steps:

1. Call them at the number provided.
2. They will send you a form requesting your name, address,

Social Security number, date of birth, income, physician information, and a list of the prescribed drugs as well as the actual prescription from your doctor.

3. After the company gets the form back, it secures the necessary forms from the appropriate drug companies, fills them out, and sends them back to you or your physician to get the necessary signatures.

4. After receipt of the signed forms, the company sends them, including your original prescription, to the drug companies.

5. The drug companies then send the medications to your doctor for you to pick up.

The company charges a one-time setup fee of $25 and an additional $10 per prescription. The $10 charge is actually a per-drug company charge. Since the company has to deal with individual drug manufacturers for various products, you are charged for dealing with each company. If you are on multiple medications, your physician, therefore, has to give you separate prescriptions for each drug but can put two or more drugs on one prescription if the same manufacturer makes them.

The Medicine Program

You can contact the Medicine Program by calling (573) 996-7300 or go to their web site at www.themedicineprogram.com.

The following steps explain how to use the Medicine Program:

1. Obtain a medication information form from the company by calling them or by downloading it from their web site.

2. Fill out the form with the patient's name, address, phone number, medication(s), and name and address of prescribing physician.

3. Mail the form and a $5 processing fee back to the company.

4. You will then receive a letter addressed to your doctor informing the doctor about the program and requesting the doctor's cooperation.

5. Read and sign your portion of the letter and forward the doctor's letter to your doctor for his or her signature.

6. After receiving all the signed papers, the company will contact the drug companies to secure your medication.

7. The medication is then sent to your physician for you to pick up.

The Medicine Program has helped thousands of individuals secure free medications from drug companies. Sometimes, however, a drug company might refuse to honor the request. In such an instance, the Medicine Program will refund the $5 dollar processing fee upon written request from the denied individual along with a copy of the letter from the drug company denying the patient's request.

Additional Information

To learn more about the drug assistance programs you can contact the individual companies, or you can call the Pharmaceutical Research and Manufacturers of American (PhRMA) at (202) 835-3400, or visit their web site at www.phrma.org.

Prescription Drugs at Low Cost

Individuals can acquire medications at a substantial discount to the retail price, in most cases, whether they have insurance or not. Using the programs described here, patients should be able to get the medication (or an equivalent substitute) at a discount and will realize significant savings, especially if they are on medications for chronic conditions. The programs described are:

- State government programs
- Generic substitution
- Brand name substitution
- Use of the Internet
- Discount pharmacy programs
- Pill cutting
- Importing drugs
- Drug company discount programs

Refer to the flow chart on page 32 to see which program is best for your situation.

State Government Programs

Various state governments have programs to assist individuals with financial difficulties in obtaining prescription drugs. These programs are needed because many people make too much money to qualify for Medicaid. These programs are different, however, from the programs that most states have to aid individuals with specific diseases or conditions that can be very expensive to manage, such as AIDS, cancer, cardiovascular disease, and diabetes.

Presently, only about half of all the states have some type of program specifically designed to aid individuals with prescription drug costs. The eligibility criteria and services provided differ from state to state and from program to program. Appendix A summarizes the state assistance programs for those states that presently offer one. States are constantly adding new programs or modifying existing ones. To keep up with all the changes and to find out the specifics for the state in which you live, log on to the web site of the National Conference of State Legislatures at www.ncsl.org/programs/health/drugaid.htm.

These programs are usually designed for seniors (persons age 65 and older) on Medicare. However, certain individuals, including those with disabilities, such as blindness, can join. Eligibility is usually based on income and this varies from state to state. These programs are usually very comprehensive, that is, they cover a lot of prescriptions.

All of the programs have some form of cost sharing, which means that the patient pays for some of the cost of the medications. These costs come in various forms like copays and deductibles. A deductible is the amount you have to spend before the program starts helping you. So if, for example, you have a deductible of $200, you will have to spend $200 on medication in that year before you can start using the program.

Some programs also have enrollment fees and some have premiums, which are amounts you pay to be in the program. Premiums are similar to what you pay to have insurance. So, in those states that have premiums, you will be charged a certain amount that you can pay over time just like you can with your car insurance.

To use the state prescription assistance program:

1. Obtain the phone number for your state's program (see appendix A for the number).
2. Get an application sent to you.
3. Enroll in the program and obtain a card.
4. Present the card at the pharmacy when filling a prescription.
5. Get the drug with a copay or at a discount.

Generic Substitution

Most people misunderstand generic drugs. The confusion has led many consumers to forego one of the most effective means of saving money when buying drugs. I will clarify some of the myths surrounding generic drugs by answering the most frequently asked questions regarding generics.

What Are Generic Drugs?

A generic drug has the same active ingredient as the brand-name drug and has been certified by the U.S. government as being equivalent to the brand-name drug. The active ingredient is the actual medicine that treats the disease. Every drug has a generic name and it usually appears in brackets after the brand name. This is the name of the active ingredient. For example, the generic name for Tylenol® is acetaminophen. You can buy the pharmacy brand of acetaminophen or acetaminophen from any other company. The ® stands for registered trademark. That means the manufacturer has a copyright protection on this name, as is the case for Tylenol.

Valium is the brand name of a drug for anxiety; diazepam is the generic name. When Valium first came out, only the brand name was available. Now other companies can manufacture the drug diazepam, since the original company no longer has exclusive rights on the drug. The other manufacturers, however, cannot call their drugs by the name Valium because that name belongs to the original manufacturer. The generic manufacturers just call it by the generic name, diazepam.

How Are Generic Drugs Different from Brand Drugs?

Although both have the same active ingredient, there are differences in the inactive ingredients chosen by the manufacturer to give the drug its bulk, change its taste, or change its look. A generic drug can, therefore, look and taste different from a brand drug. While these inactive ingredients do not change the medicine itself, some individuals might have different reactions to the various inactive ingredients. For example, one manufacturer might use a yellow dye for the color while another one uses a red dye. An individual who is allergic to a specific dye might react differently to the different drugs because of the dye. For this reason, your doctor might insist on you staying on a brand drug although a generic drug is available. Your doctor will inform your pharmacist on his or her prescription pad if this is the case. If you look at the bottom of the prescription sheet your doctor gave you, there is a little box with the letters "daw," or "dispense as written," which means the pharmacist should only give you the brand drug and not the generic.

Are Generic Drugs Safe?

For any drug to be legally sold in the United States, it must be certified by the FDA that it has met its exacting standards. Generic companies are just as regulated as manufacturers of brand drugs. Every generic drug must show not only that it is equivalent to the brand name, but also that it is manufactured in accordance with the standards set by the FDA. The manufacturer also has to show that the drug is absorbed into the human body the same way the brand drug is absorbed.

Almost 80 percent of U.S. generic drug production comes from companies that manufacture brand-name drugs using the same manufacturing facilities. The *Medical Letter,* a respected publication for physicians that reports on drugs, has stated that there have been no reports of serious differences whether a person uses a generic drug or the brand drug.

Steps for Using the Generic Substitution Technique

There are thousands of generic drugs on the market. Here are the steps you should follow to use them and save money.

1. You must get a prescription.
2. Determine if there is a generic version of the drug. (Information on available generics is offered in the chapters on the diseases. You can also ask your pharmacist.)
3. If a generic version is not available and buying the brand-name drug represents a hardship, ask your doctor for a substitute brand drug that has a generic equivalent (we will discuss brand substitution in the next section).
4. Call your doctor to inquire if you should request the generic version. If your doctor did not check the "dispense as written" box, your pharmacist may give you the generic equivalent after consulting with your doctor and, in some states, even without consulting with your doctor.

To learn more about generics, call the National Consumers League at (202) 835-3323.

Brand-Name Substitution

Healthcare professionals call brand-name substitution "therapeutic substitution." In brand-name substitution, your doctor switches you from one drug to another, both of which are used to treat the same disease. We do this ourselves, sometimes taking Motrin or Tylenol for headaches. These are different drugs, although both can be used for headaches. This is not the same as generic substitution, where you are given the same drug in an equivalent version.

Why would your doctor switch you to another drug? One reason is that usually more than one drug is approved to cure a particular disease. When a drug has been determined to treat a disease, that drug is said to be indicated for that disease. For example, Prozac has an indication for depression and a lot of people know that Prozac can treat depression. But so can drugs such as Celexa, Effexor, Paxil, and Zoloft, as well as older drugs such as Tofranil and Parnate. If you are depressed, your doctor might give you any of these drugs based on which one he or she thinks might work best for you and give you the least number of side effects. Sometimes your doctor will start you on one drug and then switch you to another one if the first one did not work, or if you develop unacceptable side effects, such as drowsiness, nausea, diarrhea, or sleeplessness.

Within a disease state, there also can be different *classes* of drugs, based on how the drugs work. For treating high blood pressure, for example, doctors have a choice of many drug classes, such as angiotensin-converting enzyme (ACE) inhibitors, calcium channel blockers, diuretics, beta-blockers, and others. Within each class, there are different drugs. So, if your doctor determines that one class is better for you than another, he or she still has choices to make within that class and can substitute one drug in the class for another.

In brand substitution you should ask your doctor if there are any less-expensive drugs that have the same indication as the drug he or she prescribed. The government has approved many different drugs as capable of treating specific medical condition, such as high blood pressure. There is a wide range of prices for these different drugs. Unless there is a compelling reason for not using a less expensive one, ask your doctor to at least start you off with a lower cost drug before going to the expensive one. The price of a drug does not indicate how good it is. A less expensive drug can be more effective for you than a more expensive one.

As an example, let us take the case of Zocor and Lescol. The government has approved both drugs to treat high cholesterol. Both are in the class of drugs called statins and work in a similar fashion. As of this writing, a 30-day supply of the starting dose of Zocor costs about $102, while Lescol costs about $42. These prices may vary depending on where you shop but the difference in cost between the two drugs is probably the same.

Using the Internet

Using the Internet to shop for prescription drugs is one of the most efficient ways to save on the cost of a prescription. It saves time, is less intrusive, and, most of the time, you can get the drug from the same pharmacy chain that you go to and still save money. Most pharmacies have web sites that sell the same medication for less, because of the savings they get from reduced rental space, smaller staff, and greater use of computers to handle operations.

There are many drug web sites, such as drugstore.com, planetrx. com, and drugemporium.com, that you might not be familiar with. If you are not comfortable dealing with these sites, there is a good chance that your own pharmacy has a site. Most of the large chains like CVS (cvs.com), Walgreen's (walgreens.com), and Eckerd Drugs (eckerd. com) have web sites that will cost less than the local pharmacy.

Purchasing pharmaceuticals through the Internet offers the following benefits:

- Lower costs than your neighborhood pharmacy.
- Shopping any time, day or night.
- Privacy.
- Home delivery of the drug.
- Most web sites provide information on various diseases.
- Most sites provide information about possible drug interactions, which happen when two drugs, if taken together, can cause bad side effects, make the medicine less effective, or even kill you. As an example, if you are taking drugs containing nitrates like nitroglycerine for your heart, you should not take Viagra. The

combination of Viagra and a nitrate drug can lead to danger-
ously low blood pressure and even death.

- Most sites have an "Ask the Pharmacists" feature that allows
  you to ask specific and personal questions to a pharmacist who
  then e-mails you the response.
- Most sites allow you to keep a history of your medications,
  which enables the pharmacy to catch any dangerous drug combinations or inappropriate medications.
- Your refills can be automated so that you don't have to remember to call in for a refill.

Internet Shopping Guidelines

The following guidelines will help make your Internet shopping experience less stressful:

- Most Internet drug sites are designed to sell you more than pharmaceuticals. This is how they make extra money. The home page
  (the screen you first see when you go to the site) is usually full
  of "deals" that are designed to attract your attention and induce
  you to buy items such as razors, toothbrushes, makeup, and the
  like. *Don't buy what you did not plan for.* This could wipe out all
  the cost savings on the medicine.
- The security of web sites is a major concern to users of the Internet. Most online drug sites are very secure and have passed rig-
  orous inspections to determine their ability to keep your
  information private and out of the reach of others. The National
  Association of Boards of Pharmacy (NABP) certifies drug web
  sites and if they pass their standards, certifies them as a Verified
  Internet Pharmacy Practice Site (VIPPS). A VIPPS seal on a site
  means that the online pharmacy has complied with the regulations of all states in which they dispense drugs.
- Be aware that while standard shipping and handling are free on
  these sites, this is true only for prescription drugs. If you order
  nonprescription items you will be charged shipping and hand-
  ing. (Some sites waive this fee if your purchase is above a certain amount.) These shipping charges can wipe out your savings.
  So to avoid shipping charges, buy only prescription drugs.
- Be wary of sites that promise to sell you drugs without a pre-

scription. Usually these sites give you an online questionnaire and based on your answers, give you a diagnosis, generate a prescription, and sell you the drug. The danger here is that the information provided might not paint a full picture of your condition that a real-life exam can. You then might end up with a drug that can harm you because of unforeseen side effects or drug interactions. In the Viagra example provided earlier, no doctor would prescribe Viagra if he or she knew you were taking a drug containing nitrates. If you left this and other information out from the questionnaire that the site provides, there is very little the site can do to protect against such dangerous combinations. These sites also are more expensive because they charge for the cost of generating a prescription.

- Stay with U.S.-based sites. There are international sites that promise to save you money by offering medications from foreign countries. It is however, difficult to assess the quality of these medications and you might be breaking the law (see the section on drug importation guidelines).

How to Use the Internet to Order Medications

Using the Internet to order medications can be easy if you follow these steps:

1. Log on to the web site and click on the pharmacy icon.
2. The first time you use the site, you will need to establish a user name and a password.
3. Most sites require you to create a patient profile, consisting of your shipping address, insurance information, and billing information.
4. Fill in the prescription request. Most sites require that you have a valid prescription for them to fulfill your request.

Web sites can get your prescription information in four ways:

1. You can mail the prescription to them.
2. They can call your doctor.
3. Your doctor can call in or fax the prescription.
4. If it is a prescription transfer from another pharmacy, the online pharmacy will call the original pharmacy to get the information.

If you provided insurance information, the pharmacy will verify your insurance eligibility and bill your insurance for the required amount and bill your credit card for the rest. The drugs are then mailed to you, usually through standard shipping at no cost, and this generally takes 7 to 12 days. Faster delivery is available for a fee.

See appendix C for a list of the most popular drug sites at the time of this writing. New sites may appear and old sites disappear with time.

Discount Pharmacy Programs

Discount pharmacy programs create savings by negotiating discount prices with various drug companies. They then pass on these savings to their members. You pay a monthly or yearly fee to join the program and you are given a card which you present at any participating pharmacy when you are filling a prescription, and you automatically receive a discounted price for the medication.

Discount pharmacies can save you money, but keep in mind the following:

- Make sure the membership fee is not too high to defeat the purpose of saving. Be especially careful with programs that charge monthly fees because although they might seem small, on a yearly basis they can be expensive and will offset any cost savings you might get from using them. Watch out also for setup fees.
- Find a program that has a large number of participating pharmacies. Be sure your neighborhood pharmacy is on the list of participating pharmacies. This is important because most discount pharmacy programs use mail order to create savings. There are times, however, when you need medication immediately and in that case you need to be able to pick up your medication at a local pharmacy.
- If the program requires that you pay a deductible when filling a prescription, be sure to add that to your membership fee to determine the total cost of participating in the program.
- Carefully examine the membership policy for any limitations on how much or how often you can use the card.
- A lot of these programs come with other benefits like savings on doctor's visits, dental work, and even legal expenses. These additional programs add to the cost of membership, so deter-

mine if you need them. If not, find a program that might not offer these additional benefits but will give you the drug program you need at a lower cost.

There are numerous pharmacy discount plans around the country. (See appendix D for a directory of some of these programs.)

Pill Cutting

A word of caution: Be sure to first seek the assistance of your doctor or pharmacist if you decide to use this technique to avoid the chance of taking the wrong dose.

Most drugs come in different dosage forms and a lot of patients are usually on the lower doses. Also, many drug companies price the different doses at roughly the same price, which means that you can actually achieve a 50 percent savings by buying a higher dose and splitting the tablet into two parts. A lot of tablets are actually scored; that is, they have marks in them that make it easier to break the tablet. If there is no scoring, pharmacies do carry pill cutters that allow you to cleanly split a tablet into two or more parts.

An example of this strategy is with the antidepressant medication Celexa, which comes in two different strengths, 20mg and 40mg scored tablets. As of this writing, a 30-day supply of 20mg Celexa costs about $65. A 30-day supply of the 40mg tablets is about $68. If you are on the 20mg dose, your doctor can prescribe the 40mg strength and then you can break it in half. You end up with a 60-day supply of the 20mg tablets and save almost 50 percent.

Guidelines Regarding Pill Cutting

Pill cutting can be an effective cost-saving strategy, but keep in mind the following:

- While most tablets can be easily split, be extra careful with tablets that are film-coated because they tend to be harder and break unevenly. Be sure to get a very sharp pill cutter to ensure clean cuts or ask your pharmacist for assistance.
- If a tablet shatters or is significantly uneven when it is split, do not take it because the chances of not receiving the correct dose are high.

- Most medicines that are labeled as *sustained release* or *extended release* have special formulations that allow them to work over a longer period of time. Most of these medications can be effectively split without affecting their mode of action. There are certain extended-release formulations, however, that should not be split because the mechanism is one that requires the pill as a whole. Examples of this type of extended-release medications that should not be split are Ditropan XL, Glucotrol XL, and Procardia XL. If you are on an extended-release medication and are not sure if it should be split, ask your pharmacist for advice.
- There are certain tablets that should not be split because the dosing regiment is designed to achieve certain levels of medications in the body. A good example of this is with birth control pills. Birth control pills are set up to deliver certain amounts of chemicals in a desired way. Do not modify this procedure because it will make the whole process ineffective.
- What if your medication is a capsule? While it is easier to deal with tablets, most capsules can be easily opened. The trick is to find out what to dilute the medication with once you open the capsule. Normally you would dissolve it in water or your favorite juice. Not all medications, however, dissolve in water and sometimes the taste can be unpleasant. Ask your pharmacist for guidance. The hope here is to put the medicine in some medium, either water, juice, or some type of sauce, and then divide the mixture to ensure that you end up with the correct amount. The other aspect to consider is storage. If you are storing the remainder for any length of time, be sure it can be stored in a way that it does not spoil or become ineffective. Always consult with your pharmacist for help.

To use the pill-cutting technique:

1. Obtain a prescription from your doctor.
2. Determine if it comes in a tablet form and at what strength. You can check with your pharmacy.
3. If there are higher strengths for the medication, ask your doctor if it is possible to get the higher strength for fewer tablets so that cutting will give you the desired quantity.
4. Ask your doctor if you can split a higher dose to get the desired

dose. If you can do that but are not exactly sure how, ask your doctor to write down clear instructions for you. Also, ask your pharmacist to assist you with the cutting if the medication is not scored and cutting it by yourself might not produce evenly split tablets.

5. Be sure to split all the medication at once so that you don't forget and end up taking more medication than is needed.

Importing Drugs

Drugs are usually much less expensive in other countries than they are in the United States even when sold by the same manufacturer who made the drug in the same manufacturing facility. This is because most countries have price controls on drugs, but the United Sates does not. In one study done in Vermont, it was found that Vermont citizens paid, on average, 81 percent higher prices for drugs compared to prices in Canada and 112 percent higher prices than in Mexico.

The reason for such price differentials is partly because Canada and Mexico impose price controls on medications and, in some cases, subsidize the cost of medicine. Because of the significant reductions in drug prices in Canada or Mexico compared with the United States, U.S. patients, especially seniors who are on multiple medications, have been known to go abroad and stock up on medicines. The FDA is concerned about this practice because of safety issues: whether the drug obtained overseas meets the same strict guidelines used in approving medications in the United States. Also, some drugs that require a prescription in this country can be obtained without prescriptions in some other countries, hence bypassing the supervision of a physician or pharmacist.

If you are thinking about trying an international drug, bear in mind:

- The FDA cannot assure the quality of a product that was not made with the procedures required by U.S. law.
- Some foreign medications may be counterfeit versions of U.S.-approved medicine, which makes them illegal.
- If you have a bad reaction to a drug that is not well known in the United States, treatment may be delayed or hindered because of lack of knowledge about the drug.

- It may be against some state and federal laws to possess certain medicines without a prescription.

Guidelines for Drug Importation

The FDA has issued some guidelines to be used in dealing with the issue of importing drugs. The FDA considers any imported drug an unapproved drug if it was not manufactured in accordance with FDA guidelines and certified as such by the FDA. (This also applies to foreign-made versions of U.S.-approved drugs.) The possessor of the drug then has to prove that the drug is an approved drug.

This does not mean that you cannot bring foreign or unapproved drugs into the United States. To bring in a foreign or unapproved drug you must follow these guidelines:

- The product has to be for personal use and not for commercial purposes. To ensure that it is for personal use, the amount has to be for about a three-month supply. You may be allowed more than a three-month supply if you can prove that you need more than that to treat your disease.
- You must show that the product will be used for its intended use. To accomplish this, all you need to do is affirm in writing that you will use the product for its intended use and provide the name and address of the doctor licensed in the United States who will be responsible for your treatment. You may also provide evidence that the drug is for the continuation of treatment started in a foreign country. A note from the doctor who gave you the prescription in the foreign country might be sufficient.
- Make sure that there is some type of identification or label that identifies the medicine you are carrying.
- Do not lie or misrepresent what you are carrying since this might arouse suspicion about whether the drug is lawful.

These rules for bringing in drugs also apply to importing drugs by mail and using foreign-based web sites.

Be aware of travel costs. If you go to a foreign country just to buy drugs, you have to add the cost of travel, which includes transportation, lodging, and meals. If this cost is significant, it might defeat the whole cost-saving idea.

Drug Company Discount Programs

With the growing debate over lack of prescription coverage for seniors, several drug companies have created programs that allow individuals on Medicare to buy their drugs at a discount. In all of these programs, the individual must be covered by Medicare, have no source of prescription drug coverage, and meet certain income limits. As of this writing four companies have announced the details of their programs: GlaxoSmithKline, Lilly, Novartis, and Pfizer.

GlaxoSmithKline issues the Orange Card, through which a senior can obtain any GlaxoSmithKline drug at a 25 percent discount on the retail price. The income limits in 2002 were $30,000 for singles and $40,000 for couples (in Alaska the limits were $33,000 for singles and $44,000 for couples). To reach the Glaxo program, call (888) ORANGE6 (888-672-6436).

The Lilly program is called Lilly Answers. The income limits in 2002 were $18,000 for singles and $24,000 for couples. With the Lilly program, any qualifier pays a flat fee of $12 for a 30-day supply of any Lilly drug except controlled substances. To reach the Lilly program, call (877) RX-LILLY (800-795-4559).

The Novartis program is called the CareCard. This program has the same criteria as the Glaxo program, promising a 30 percent discount on the retail price of the company's drugs. To reach the CareCard program, call (866) 974-CARE (866-974-2273).

Pfizer's Share Card program has the same income criteria as Lilly's program ($18,000 per single and $24,000 per couple). The qualifier pays a flat fee of $15 for a 30-day supply of any Pfizer drug. Through its Share Card program, Pfizer also offers access to health education literature and referral services. To reach the Pfizer program, call (800) 717-6005.

These programs are relatively new and continue to evolve. Abbott, AstraZeneca, Aventis, Bristol-Myers Squibb, and Johnson and Johnson joined Glaxo and Novartis to offer one program called the Together Rx Card. The eligibility criteria are seniors on Medicare with no drug coverage and income levels of less than $28,000 for singles and less than $35,000 for couples.

PART THREE

Other Areas of Healthcare Cost

CHAPTER 6

Physician Services

P hysicians get paid for the time they spend taking your history and examining you, and for performing various diagnostic tests and procedures like surgeries. The most expensive aspects are the procedures. Your primary care physician (PCP), who could be a family doctor, general practitioner, internist, pediatrician, or OB/GYN, spends more time talking with you and less time performing procedures, while the specialist (with the notable exception of the psychiatrist) spends less time talking to you and more time performing procedures. This is why specialists cost more to visit than PCPs. The more the specialists you interact with, the more expensive your medical bill will be.

So, if you have been advised to have a procedure, be sure that it is necessary. Why? Because procedures bring in more revenue and some doctors may perform a lot of them unnecessarily just to increase their income. Also, procedures do carry risks and you might end up with complications that are not warranted. Get at least one more opinion, or even a third one if it is a complicated procedure or if you are just not sure.

Paying for Physician Services When You Have Insurance Coverage

When you have HMO coverage, your physician visits are covered by your copay, which can range from $5 to $20. That is all you pay, assuming that you visit the PCP that is designated in your plan. Your copay will also cover the tests that the physician performs in his or her office, such as a blood test, urinalysis, EKG (heart exam), or X ray. If any of these tests have to be performed outside the physician's office, you are still covered and will not incur any additional costs as long as your PCP is the one who authorized the test. If you have to see a specialist, you will also pay only a copay as long as your PCP referred you to the specialist and the specialist is in the plan network. If you visit a specialist *without* a referral from your PCP, even if that specialist is in the network, the insurance company will not cover it.

In an HMO plan, the physician has already agreed to the fee schedule and cannot charge the patient any more than the insurance will pay. In fact, the patient has no paperwork to deal with and except for the office visit copay, has nothing else to do in term of the charges. However, the whole system falls apart if you have to see a physician outside the network. A lot of insurance companies will not cover out-of-network visits except for emergency situations.

If you have an indemnity plan, you can visit whichever physician you want but the company will pay only a percentage, usually 80 percent of what is deemed usual and customary. Physicians have all the control in terms of how much they can charge. The insurance company decides how much it wants to pay and the patient has to pay for the rest. There is a lot of paperwork to contend with and the patient usually ends up spending a lot of money out of pocket, whether he or she is seeing a PCP or a specialist. A patient concerned about the cost of a physician visit who has indemnity insurance should therefore inquire ahead of time how much the visit will cost. Work out a financial plan in advance by talking to the doctor and office staff to get a firm estimate of the treatment cost.

One way to reduce your physician fees even with insurance is to use the phone. Every time you visit a physician for care, you are charged a copay or your share of the indemnity insurance. Many times these visits are to seek comfort when dealing with a chronic illness or just to ask some questions. Some of these questions can be handled over the phone and your physician can determine if you actually need to come in. Do not abuse this privilege, however. If you get into the habit of constantly calling your physician for every little issue and then keeping him or her on the phone for long periods of time, the physician may start ignoring you or actually charge you for the phone consult.

The most important aspect in managing the cost of physician services is to understand what is covered and what is not covered, as specified in your insurance manual. Remember, your policy is a contract. If a service was not part of that contract, it is nearly impossible to get the company to pay for it. If you have any doubt about a service, call the company ahead of time to get clarification and if they say it is covered, get a written notice to that effect. This way if it has to go to arbitration or a court, you have a document to back you up.

Handling the Cost of Physician Services If You Do Not Have Insurance

If you do not have insurance that covers physician services, you should be thinking of how to get the services for free or at a reduced rate.

Sources of Free Care

There are various establishments that provide free physician services. These include schools, job sites, medical university centers, and community centers.

Many schools have health centers where any member of that establishment can go in and get a checkup for free. While some of these centers do not provide very comprehensive care, they provide decent enough care that might be sufficient for the needs of the individual.

A lot of employers also have health centers at their job sites. Some employers who do not provide health insurance for their workers do provide a facility for employees to get routine care and immunizations. These centers can handle some of the basic healthcare needs and follow-up care.

While medical university centers do not routinely provide free services, they are involved in medical studies and are always looking for volunteers. As part of getting involved in a study, you will be given a thorough physical exam and workup, for free. It is important to note, however, that this is not recommended as a way to get routine care, since this method provides no continuity of care—when the study is over, you have to move on or find another study. Also, medical studies, while a necessary part of medicine, carry risks. Be sure you thoroughly understand what you are getting into and are fully informed of the risks involved.

Community centers and churches often hold health fairs where physicians perform various services for free to the community. Again, while this might be a good short-term solution especially for those who have not been to a doctor in a while and might be worried about a condition but do not know where to start, it is still necessary to establish a long-term relationship with a physician or health center.

Physician Services at Reduced Fees

In trying to save on the cost of physician services, it is always good to remember that specialists charge more than generalists, so the more specialized the physician, the greater the chance of the fees being on the high side. To any extent possible, stay with PCPs, especially general and family physicians, because they cost less than internists. So first call around and inquire about their rates. Also inquire about payment plans. If you are afraid that the doctor might not agree to a plan ahead of time, visit the doctor and get the help you need. After that, tell him or her you can't pay but would like to arrange for a payment plan. As long as you stick to the plan, you are not going to be sent to a credit collector. However, do this only when you are really desperate and need to see a doctor.

There are other options available to get physician services at reduced costs. Congress passed the Emergency Medical Treatment and Active Labor Act (EMTALA) in 1986 to ensure that no one goes untreated in the face of an emergency. This law requires emergency rooms to treat any individual regardless of ability to pay. This means that once a person shows up at an emergency room he or she cannot be turned away because of lack of insurance.

Another option for individuals without health insurance is to use federally funded health clinics. There are almost 4,000 sites in all 50 states that provide services to the underserved. Because these clinics receive federal grants, they cannot refuse to treat a patient because of lack of insurance. These clinics represent valuable sources of primary care for many low-income patients and are becoming actively involved in Medicaid Managed Care programs. To determine if a clinic in your area is federally funded, call the Health Resources and Services Administration (HRSA) at (800) 400-2742.

It is important to be able to communicate openly and trustingly with your physician, and this includes talking to him or her about the cost of any medical intervention. For those who are embarrassed to talk to their doctor about the cost of treatment, it may be comforting to know that the American Medical Association states the following in its Fundamental Elements of the Patient-Physician Relationship:

The patient has the right to receive information from physicians and to discuss the benefits, risks, and costs of appropriate treatment alternatives. Patients should receive guidance from their physicians as to the optimal course of action. Patients are also entitled to obtain copies or summaries of their medical records, to have their questions answered, to be advised of potential conflicts of interest that their physicians might have, and to receive independent professional opinions.

CHAPTER 7

Institutional Care

Hospitals and Nursing Homes

A s you will recall from the healthcare cost pyramid on page 6, this is the most expensive aspect of healthcare cost. So everybody should do what it takes not to need hospital or nursing home care, or at least to reduce the amount of time spent in these institutions. We do have the power to prevent or minimize the things that land us in hospitals or nursing homes.

Hospitals

There are three reasons you end up in a hospital: emergency care, urgent care, and elective care.

An emergency is where a serious medical condition arises suddenly and without warning, for example, a crushing chest pain that might indicate a heart attack. Any sudden change in a person's condition should be considered an emergency. In these situations, call 911.

Urgent care is when you have a problem for which you would normally go to your doctor, but the problem occurs after your doctor's office is closed and you feel you can't wait until the office is open again. With urgent care you can usually drive yourself to the hospital, or a family member, friend, or neighbor can take you there. Certain facilities operate in a manner between a hospital and a doctor's office. You can't stay there overnight, but they are open 24 hours with doctors available to handle problems related to urgent care. They are known as urgicenters and treat individuals on a drop-in basis. Urgicenters handle minor problems and perform a lot of primary care. Other centers perform urgent care that requires procedures. These facilities, known as ambulatory surgical centers or surgicenters, perform minor surgeries like hernia repairs and cosmetic surgeries. Again, in all of these centers, the patient gets to go home the same day.

Elective care is when you need a procedure done that requires the facilities of a hospital but the procedure doesn't have to be done immediately. Elective care requires scheduling a date for the procedure. There is a lot of preprocedure planning that involves meeting with several members of the team who will be responsible for your care. A good example of an elective procedure is hip-replacement surgery. Usually this requires prior consultation with your primary care physician and the orthopedic surgeon or surgeons who will perform the procedure. During this preprocedure stage, you are told what to expect, the risks involved, and any alternatives that might be available. Most cosmetic surgeries are elective procedures.

Inpatient vs. Outpatient Care

All hospital care is classified as either inpatient or outpatient care. Inpatient care means that the patient stays overnight in the hospital for one or more days. With outpatient care, the patient is treated or a procedure performed and the patient gets to go home the same day.

It is important to know if a hospital visit will be on an inpatient or outpatient basis because the number of days spent in the hospital plays a significant role in the overall cost of your hospital care. Also keep in mind that many patients who are in the hospital on an inpatient basis may end up with unnecessary procedures. Procedures account for a huge portion of the hospital bill.

Choosing a Hospital

All hospitals can be placed in one of four categories: community hospital, public hospital, university hospital, or specialty hospital.

Community hospitals are usually small hospitals with fewer than 500 beds. They provide patient care for the most common conditions affecting individuals in the community. They usually are not involved in research. The appeal of community hospitals is that they are small and can give you more timely care, and they are usually located close by so that they are easy to get to, and visits from friends and family are easier. Community hospitals can be for-profit or nonprofit.

Public hospitals are owned and operated by the government—federal, state or city. These include such hospitals as the Veterans Affairs hospitals. Because the government subsidizes them, they are usually less expensive and so are a source of good care for less money. However, they can be more crowded than community hospitals. Some public hospitals also affiliate themselves with universities and so serve as teaching hospitals.

University hospitals are basically teaching hospitals. They are designed to train doctors from medical school through residency, the training that occurs after medical school, to specialization. They may have thousands of beds and may be spread out over large areas, sometimes even in different cities. Their services range from simple primary care to very complex procedures like brain surgery. The advantage of university hospitals is that they usually have experts on many disease conditions and can handle very complex cases. These centers, however, can be very crowded and patients may sometimes feel that the care is impersonal since many doctors might see them and their cases may be discussed among students and other doctors for teaching purposes. (It is important to know that you have the right not to have your case discussed to teach students.) University hospitals can be owned by the government or be private and for-profit.

Specialty hospitals are designed to focus on one condition. They are usually very research-oriented and are on the cutting edge of the management of that disease. An example of a specialty hospital is Memorial Sloan Kettering Cancer Center in New York City, where the focus is on the treatment of cancer. Specialty hospitals are usually teaching hospitals. The advantage of a specialty hospital is that you will likely meet with experts in the field of that disease who know the latest advances in the treatment of that condition and so are suited for dealing with very complex cases or with those that have failed to respond to conventional therapy. Specialty hospitals, however, are very expensive. Also, because they are research-oriented, patients are likely going to be recruited for clinical studies, which you can refuse to take part in.

In choosing a hospital, you should work with your primary care physician to determine which one is appropriate for you. This assumes, however, that you have the time to plan for a hospital visit. (In an emergency, the emergency personnel largely decide the choice of your hospital.) While your PCP should be an important consultant in your choice of hospital, the final say is yours. In that regard, there are three criteria you should consider before picking one: expertise, convenience, and cost.

Expertise relates to the ability of the hospital to manage your condition effectively. Routine care or procedures can be effectively managed by all the different types of hospitals. If you have a more complex situation, such as needing open-heart surgery, you want to know if the hospital has expertise in that area. Expertise is usually assessed by the number of cases per year that the hospital handles in that particular condition. Several studies have shown that the hospitals that handle high volumes of a particular condition have the lowest cases of things going wrong. You can find out how a hospital rates for a particular procedure by looking at the "Quality Check" report for that hospital produced by the Joint Commission on Accreditation of Healthcare Organizations (JCAHO), an independent nonprofit organization that evaluates and accredits hospitals and other healthcare facilities. Log onto their web site at www.jcaho.org to see how your hospital is rated.

Convenience has to do not only with how easy it is to get to the hospital, but also how you are treated once you are there, not in the medical sense but with respect to your time and level of respect. No matter the expertise of the hospital, if you have to wait hours before being seen or you have to put up with condescending and disrespectful behavior from the hospital staff, it might not be very helpful to your state of mind. Your state of mind and how you feel about yourself can be very powerful in your recovery. If you have to travel a longer distance just to avoid long waits and disrespectful attitudes, then you should.

Managing the Cost of Hospitalization

As of this writing, the average hospital stay is five days and costs over $11,000. To understand why hospitals are very expensive, it is necessary to realize that hospitals provide essentially two services: a hotel service and a medical service. While these two operations work hand in hand to ensure your care, financially they are distinct systems.

The president or chief executive officer (CEO) of the hospital, while technically responsible for everything in the hospital, is largely running the hotel aspect of the hospital. Every aspect of your hospital care outside what the doctors do, from your room to the food to the medications to the nursing care to the tests, are in this category. Hospitals have very large overheads and large staffs, a lot of whom perform clerical and administrative functions.

The medical service is usually under the direction of the chief medical officer. In hospitals, most of the doctors are usually not employed by the hospital. The hospital gives them "admitting privileges," meaning that they can have their patients use the hospital facility for their care or for the doctors to perform various procedures. The doctors do not pay the hospital for this privilege. You are billed separately for the services rendered by the doctor and the services rendered by the "hotel." Every doctor who interacts with you in the hospital gives you a bill for his or her services. So, every time a doctor is brought in for consultation on your case, you receive a charge.

Over half of all hospital bills go to the government in the form of Medicare and Medicaid billings. Private insurance gets about a third. Because the government pays for so much of the hospital bill, it developed a system to get a handle on the cost. This system classifies diseases into categories called Diagnostic-Related Groups (DRGs). For each group, the government determines the average length of stay and cost of treatment. It then pays the hospital a given amount for those illnesses no matter how long it took for the hospital to treat the patient. This resulted in hospitals cutting back on the number of days patients stayed in the hospital. The DRG guidelines even determine which conditions do not warrant hospital stays. So if a patient is admitted to the hospital for a condition for which the DRG has determined that no hospital stay is needed, the hospital does not get paid. Such conditions are expected to be handled on an outpatient basis.

Nearly every individual ends up being billed for some portion of his or her hospital stay. Insurance companies pay a percentage of the charges and the hospital bills the patient for the rest. There are no laws that tell the hospitals how much they can charge for a particular care or procedure, so charges for the same services vary widely from hospital to hospital even in the same area. As a general rule, public hospitals charge the least, followed by community hospitals, then university hospitals, with specialty hospitals charging the most. For those interested in seeing how prices can vary, log onto the web site of the American Hospital Directory (www.ahd.com). The AHD compiles data from more than 6,000 hospitals and tells you how much each hospital bills for a particular condition and the average length of stay for patients with that condition. It also shows you how that compares with the national average.

Dealing with Hospital Costs If You Have Insurance

If you have insurance in any form—HMO, Medicaid, Medicare, indemnity, and so on—you must understand that the insurance company is likely not going to cover everything the hospital bills you for. The first place to start, therefore, is to look at your policy to determine what is covered and what is not. These are the questions you need answered:

- If the insurance is managed care insurance, is the hospital part of the plan's network? Network hospitals have negotiated rates with the plan and you will be covered for a lot of the hospital's charges based on your policy. If the hospital is not in the network, you will have to pay for all or a big portion of the charges, unless the visit was due to an emergency. With Medicare and Medicaid, the hospital just has to be certified as a Medicare or Medicaid provider for you to get the benefits (nearly all hospitals are). With indemnity insurance, you can go to any hospital of your choosing but remember the plan will only pay a portion of the charges that it determines to be usual and customary. Also remember the caps on your insurance. If you exceed that cap, you are responsible for 100 percent of the charges.
- What aspects of the "hotel" and "medical" charges are covered? Your insurance plan does not give you free reign to ask for five-star services. If your plan pays only for a shared room and you ask for a private room, you will be charged for the difference. This applies to other services that you request outside the customary services, for example, asking for a special diet.

In looking at the "medical" aspect of your bill, be sure that you follow your plan's protocol. In an HMO plan, for example, you should be admitted to a network hospital by your PCP or a specialist to whom you were referred by your PCP. While in the hospital, be sure that consultations are done with your PCP's approval and/or the doctors are all affiliated with the hospital and are in the plan's network. While this might sound cumbersome and difficult to handle especially if you are very sick, it might mean the difference between coming out financially unscathed and having to file for bankruptcy. If you can't handle it, find a friend or family member to help you with this. Remember, procedures that physicians perform account for the bulk of hospital charges, so handle this aspect with all seriousness.

Dealing with Hospital Costs If You Do Not Have Health Insurance

If you do not have insurance, do everything you can to stay away from the hospital. In an emergency you may not have a choice, but if it is an urgent or elective procedure, investigate the possibility of using an urgicenter or surgicenter before using the hospital. If you have to use a hospital, look at government hospitals first, then community hospitals, then university hospitals, and specialty hospitals last. If you end up in a hospital, remember that no hospital can turn you away for treatment especially if it is an emergency. Keep the following in mind in dealing with hospital costs if you do not have insurance:

- The first thing to do if you need hospitalization, especially for an elective procedure where you can plan ahead, is to determine if you qualify for any insurance program. Are you poor enough to qualify for Medicaid? Are there any government programs that can give you assistance? Call your state health office (see appendix A for phone numbers) to find out. Do you belong to a group through which you can get some form of health coverage? Do these things before you get into the hospital because if you do them after, even if you get the insurance, it might not cover a cost that was incurred prior to your getting the coverage.
- Always get a second or third opinion about any procedure. Many treatments have alternatives and sometimes you might not even need the procedure at all. Be sure, however, that you do not stay away from a treatment because of the cost, but rather because another well-respected professional determined that it is not necessary.
- Check out government-run clinics and hospitals. These establishments are not only less expensive but will charge you based on your income, that is, on a sliding scale, and will work out payment plans that you can live with.
- Check out the Hill-Burton Free Care program, a federal program for

people without insurance whose incomes fall within certain poverty guidelines. Certain facilities have contracted with the government to provide free care to those who qualify. It is not an insurance program and can only be used after you have used the service or you can apply when you know you will use the service. You do not have to be a U.S. citizen to use the program but you must have been in the country for at least three months. To find out if you qualify or which facilities in your area are part of the plan, call (800) 638-0742 or log on to www.hrsa.gov/osp/dfcr.

- The government subsidizes most hospitals, especially teaching hospitals, because they are expected to take care of individuals who cannot pay for what the hospital charges. In these cases, the hospital will charge you on a sliding scale based on income and you can negotiate a payment plan.
- If you have a complicated or rare disease, one that in all likelihood is very expensive to treat, look into participating in clinical trials. In clinical trials, all your expenses will be paid for including, in some cases, your transportation. Be sure you understand what will be done and realize that if it is what is known as a double-blind trial, you might not be getting the active treatment but might be getting a fake treatment or placebo and neither you nor your doctor will know until the end. Not all studies are double blind, however. Some are known as open trials, where you and your doctor know exactly what you are getting. As in all cases with studies, do not sign the form agreeing to it until you understand all the risks involved. If you are not sure, get someone else to review it for you. To find out more about what trials are going on, call the National Institutes of Health at (800) 411-1222 or log on to their web site at www.clinicaltrials.gov.
- Avoid unnecessary services like private rooms and special meals if you can.
- If you need medication that can be brought in from the outside, like Tylenol or even some prescription drugs, it might be cheaper to get them from an outside pharmacy than from the hospital pharmacy. Discuss this with your doctor and let the nurses help you with the medication regimens.
- Discuss any consultations with other doctors ahead of time and be sure they are absolutely needed so you don't end up with more physician charges than are necessary.

• When you get the bill, go over it with a fine-tooth comb. Very few patients do and there have been stories of hospitals charging exorbitant amounts sometimes for services that were not even rendered. You should realize that all bills are negotiable. Start by getting a sense of what the hospital charges the government for that service. You can get that information from the AHD web site (www.ahd.com). Then negotiate from there. When you have reached a satisfactory amount, you can work out a payment plan with the hospital that you can live with.

What to Do If You Have Disputes with the Hospital

Many patients find their hospital bills incomprehensible and despite their best efforts to clarify things with the hospital are still not satisfied. A number of organizations help patients deal with disputes related to hospital care.

A good place to start is with your local chamber of commerce. Call and ask if there are any local patient advocacy groups. Many areas have patient advocacy groups that will act on the patients' behalf to resolve issues related to their care. One such group is the Patient Advocacy Coalition in Denver (www.patientadvocacy.net) that represents patients who have disputes with their insurance plans.

The Medical Care Ombudsman Program (MCOP) reviews disputes between patients and health plans, especially in cases of denials, with the help of an independent panel of experts. They work in all states and their findings are usually binding. They can be reached at (888) 313-6267 or www.mcman.com.

Nursing Homes

About 11 percent of all patients discharged from hospitals end up in nursing homes. A nursing home is like a hospital serving the "hotel" and "medical" functions. In nursing homes, more emphasis is placed on the hotel function and not as much on the medical function as in the hospital. While the hospital bill is mostly from the medical function, the nursing home bill is largely from the hotel services.

There are three types of nursing homes providing various degrees of medical care:

- Residential-care facilities (RCFs)
- Intermediate-care facilities (ICFs)
- Skilled-nursing facilities (SNFs)

In RCFs, the residents are assisted with their activities of daily living such as meals and grooming. They are monitored for any medical conditions and are given simple and routine medical care if needed. RCFs are suited for those who are not really that ill but do not want to live at home alone and do not want to deal with the daily chores of housekeeping. Some of these facilities are also called assisted living facilities.

ICFs have more medical care functions than RCFs. In addition to the functions provided in RCFs, ICFs provide regular nursing care, although not on a 24-hour basis. They can also provide more recreational facilities and other services like rehabilitation care and physical therapy.

SNFs are the most medically intense of all the nursing home facilities. They provide 24-hour nursing care and are more closely monitored by the government.

Choosing a Nursing Home

There are several things to take into account before deciding which nursing home to choose:

- How good is the medical care at the nursing home? This consideration depends in part on how much medical care is needed. If you are in relatively good health, then an RCF or ICF will be sufficient. If more intensive care is needed, then an SNF should be chosen. If the patient is coming out of a hospital, most likely he or she would be sent to an SNF. Some state laws require that a hospital cannot allow an elderly person who is unable to take care of himself or herself to go home unless an adequate plan for care has been established.
- Nursing homes have their own doctors to monitor and care for their residents and some homes prefer that their doctors be the ones administering medical care. Since the patient's doctor might know more about the patient than the nursing home's doctor, be sure that the nursing home allows the patient's own private doctor to visit the patient.
- Find out about the certification of the nursing home. Call your local health office, the state health office, or Medicare to inquire about

the track record of any nursing home you are interested in. Local consumer groups focused on elder care can also help you in this regard. While nursing homes are not required to be certified, certification is important because most insurance, including government insurance like Medicaid and Medicare, will not reimburse a nursing home for any service if it is not certified. Certification also means that the government more closely monitors the nursing home.

- Visit the home and get a feel for what the home provides. What does it look like? Is it clean? Do the residents look happy? Talk to the workers and residents themselves and ask them what they think. Ask the workers how long they have been there. If there is a lot of worker turnover, it might not be a good place to be.
- While the administrators of the home will give you a tour of the facility, be sure to schedule a tour of your own, preferably unannounced, to get a real-life feel for what the home offers.
- Inquire about the long-term goals of the home. Because of reimbursement issues, a lot of nursing homes are cutting back on long-term care and increasing their acute care services. What this means is that the hotel functions like meals, grooming, and physical and rehabilitation programs are being short-changed and the medical functions of taking care of the sick are being emphasized. These nursing homes are moving toward becoming, in essence, hospitals.

Managing the Cost of Nursing Homes

Some estimates currently put the cost of nursing home care from $25,000 to as high as $50,000 a year, with the average being about $38,000. Medicare pays about 15 percent of the cost with Medicaid covering 43 percent, private insurance paying for 14.5 percent, and individuals responsible for the other 37.5 percent. Many individuals are under the mistaken belief that Medicare covers nursing home care. Medicare is an acute care insurance program. It will only cover a portion of nursing home care under the following conditions:

- Medicare pays only for stays in SNFs that are certified by Medicare. So be sure the facility is an SNF that is a Medicare-accredited.
- Your medical condition caused you to stay in a hospital for at least three days before entering the home.

- You entered the SNF within 30 days of having been discharged from the hospital.
- A doctor or another certified health professional determined that your condition requires you to stay in an SNF.
- Medicare covers only medical services and not custodial services like meals and grooming.
- Medicare pays for services for the first 20 days and for days 21 through 100, you have to pay a copay of $97 (in year 2000). Medicare supplemental insurance can cover this copay, but after day 100, you pay for all your services. If you have HMO Medicare, ask your plan for its nursing home coverage. Most of them follow the traditional Medicare policy stated above.

Medicaid is a more generous program and pays for the lion's share of the nursing home. Medicaid will cover not only the medical care but also the custodial services. To be eligible for Medicaid coverage, you have to meet certain income and asset criteria, that is, you have to have limited income and assets. If you are not already poor, you must exhaust all your assets before Medicaid can assist you. Medicaid rules vary from state to state and can be very complex. There are rules that govern what an asset is and which ones are counted in deciding how many assets you have. There are also laws on how much asset you can transfer to your spouse and the conversion of eligible to noneligible assets. The best thing to do is consult with a financial planner who is well versed in your state's Medicaid program to help you determine how you can qualify for Medicaid coverage for nursing home care.

Two other strategies for managing nursing home costs besides qualifying for Medicaid are long-term care insurance and using alternatives to nursing home care.

Long-Term Insurance

Because a substantial part of nursing home costs is borne by individuals, many financial planners advise that it is prudent to buy long-term care insurance. Remember that just because you have health insurance, it does not mean that you have nursing home coverage. They are different. Meet with a financial planner or call your insurance agent to figure out what plan is good for you. Remember, the younger you are, the less expensive the premium. Some financial planners recommend getting long-term insurance at age 55. Your planner should ensure that the plan is highly rated, has been around for at least 10 years, and covers nearly all the things you will need in a nursing home. A good place to start is by calling the Health Insurance Counseling and Advocacy Program (HICAP), an advocacy group that helps seniors with Medicare and other health issues. The phone number is (800) 434-0222.

Alternatives to Nursing Homes

While a lot of individuals end up in nursing homes, there are many who would prefer to stay in their own homes and receive the care they need. Medicare offers two programs for certain beneficiaries who need comprehensive medical care and social services:

- Program for All-Inclusive Care for the Elderly (PACE)
- Social Health Maintenance Organizations (SHMOs)

PACE

PACE is a comprehensive program that provides medical care by doctors, nurses, and other health professionals at the home of the individual, avoiding the need to go to a hospital or nursing home. PACE provides social services, drugs, nursing facility care, restorative therapies, personal care, supportive therapies, and meals. If transportation is needed, that is also provided. The services can also be provided at an adult health center or in-patient facility. PACE is a combined Medicare-Medicaid program, hence individuals must meet eligibility criteria for both Medicare and their state's Medicaid program. As of this writing there are eighteen states with PACE activity or approved PACE providers: California, Colorado, Florida, Kansas, Maryland, Massachusetts, Michigan, Missouri, New Mexico, New York, Ohio, Oregon, Pennsylvania, South Carolina, Tennessee, Texas, Washington, and Wisconsin.

Other criteria included for eligibility to join PACE are:

- You must be at least 55 years old.
- You must live in a PACE service area.
- You must be screened by a team of doctors, nurses, and other health professionals.
- You must sign and agree to the terms of the enrollment agreement.

SHMOs

An SHMO is offered by an HMO to provide the full range of benefits offered by the HMO but with the addition of chronic care benefits, and full range of home- and community-based services such as homemaker, respite care, and medical transportation. Membership offers health benefits that are provided by Medicare or other senior plans. As of this writing, only four plans provide SHMO services:

- Kaiser Permanente in Portland, Oregon
- SCAN in Long Beach, California
- Elderplan in Brooklyn, New York
- Health Plan of Nevada in Las Vegas, Nevada

Other Alternatives to Nursing Homes

Additional alternatives include:

- Elder Care Locator, a program that can assist you in finding necessary and convenient elder facilities in your area. The phone number is (800) 677-1116.
- Community and home care programs that provide assistance to seniors living at home with such services as Meals on Wheels, friendly visiting and shopping services, and adult daycare facilities. Check with your local department of aging.

Resources

American Association of Homes
and Services for the Aging
(202) 783-2242
www.aasha.org

Assisted Living Facilities of
America
(703) 691-1116

Centers for Medicare and Medicaid
Services (Formerly HCFA)
(800) MEDICARE
(800-633-4227)
www.medicare.gov

National Citizens Coalition for
Nursing Home Reform
(202) 332-7424

National Long-term Care
Resource Center
(612) 624-5434

CHAPTER 8

Employment and Family Issues

W hen you get sick, you worry about getting well again. Unfortunately, with many diseases, especially chronic illnesses, you come to realize that the illness might never go away and you start thinking about what this means for the rest of your life. Two areas that are significantly affected by illnesses are employment and family relationships. The financial and emotional impact can be huge. In this chapter we will examine the costs involved in these areas, some of which can be measured and some of which cannot.

Employment

One of the areas that may be affected is your ability to earn a living through working. Some of the questions that you might be asking are:

- How does my illness affect the way I do my job?
- How does my employer view my illness?
- Can I be denied a job because I have a particular illness?
- What protections do I have if my employer penalizes me because of my illness?

The answers to these questions are based on laws, both federal and state. You should, therefore, seek the help of a legal professional who is familiar with employment laws. This chapter will provide you with some basic knowledge on employment laws related to health and what your rights are. Be sure to consult with expert legal help before making any decisions on these matters.

Your rights to have your employer make reasonable accommodations for you when you have a health problem are based on three federal laws:

- The Americans with Disability Act (ADA)
- The Rehabilitation Act
- The Family Medical Leave Act (FMLA)

The Americans with Disability Act (ADA)

The ADA is a federal law passed in 1990 that extends civil rights protection to individuals with physical or mental disabilities. Title 1 of the law makes it illegal for employers to discriminate against employees or individuals seeking employment on the basis of their disability. The actual law states:

> No *covered entity* shall discriminate against a *qualified individual* with a *disability* because of the disability of such individual in regard to job application procedures, the hiring, advancement, or discharge of employees, employee compensation, job training, and other terms, and conditions, and privileges of employment [emphasis added].

The law further requires that employers make *reasonable accommodations* to the known physical or mental limitations of the individual unless such accommodations would impose *undue hardship* on the business. It is important to define some of the terms because they are critical as to who is covered under this law and what protections are provided.

Covered Entity

Any private employer with more than 15 employees is covered under this law. All public employees except those of the federal government are also covered. The law also covers labor unions and religious organizations. Besides the federal government, Native American tribes and tax-exempt private membership clubs also are not covered. The covered entity may not discriminate in any aspects of a job, including pay, promotions, training, firing, and hiring, as well as leave benefits.

Qualified Individual

A qualified individual is a person with a disability who has the skills, experience, education, or other qualifications required by a job. The person must be able to perform the essential functions of that job with or without reasonable accommodations. The term "essential functions" is key because if a particular task is not needed as part of the main job, then it not an essential function.

Disability

The definition of disability under the ADA is met when these three things occur:

1. The individual has a substantial impairment, either physical or mental, that limits one or more major life activities. Major life activities include hearing, seeing, speaking, walking, breathing, performing manual tasks, maintaining social relationships, learning, and ability to take care of oneself. The disability must be one that cannot be corrected by medications or other means.
2. The individual is regarded as having a substantial impairment. This is met if an employer, prospective employer or other individuals treat the person as having an impairment, even if he or she does not have one.
3. The individual has a history of disability. If someone shows that he or she had a medical condition but no longer has it, an employer cannot use that against the person. For example, if someone was an alcoholic or a drug abuser but is not currently abusing, an employer or prospective employer cannot discriminate based on that. The ADA does not, however, bar an employer from conducting drug testing on employees or prospective employees for current drug use.

Reasonable Accommodations

A reasonable accommodation is a change in the job or workplace to enable the person with a disability to perform a job. It also means making the changes that would allow the person with a disability to enjoy the same privileges that all the other employees enjoy. Employers are not expected to lower the quality or quantity standard expected of the job.

Undue Hardship

Reasonable accommodation should not cause undue hardship to an employer. Undue hardship is defined as "an action requiring significant difficulty or expense." This takes into account the size and resources of the employer. What constitutes undue hardship to a small employer might not be a hardship to a large employer.

Other Things to Remember about the ADA

The following should also be taken into account with regard to the ADA:

- If you are seeking a job, the prospective employer cannot ask you if you have a disability. The employer can, however, inquire whether you can do the job with or without reasonable accommodations.
- An employer cannot require you to take a medical examination before offering you a job. The employer can, however, ask you to demonstrate how you can do the job with or without reasonable accommodation. After you are hired, or have been offered the job, the employer can require you to take a physical exam or other medical tests. This requirement must be one that is imposed on all new employees for that job category. If your test reveals a disability, an employer cannot reject you unless he or she can prove that the disability would prevent you from performing the essential duties of the job with or without reasonable accommodation.
- An employer cannot perform medical tests on employees unless such tests are directly related to the job function. There has to be a legitimate business reason for such a test, otherwise it would be considered arbitrary and hence illegal under the ADA. Testing for current use of illegal drugs is legal under the ADA.
- The ADA does not specify which diseases are covered. It does, however, specify diseases that are not covered. They include kleptomania (compulsive stealing), pyromania (setting fires), compulsive gambling, and all sexual behaviors. Because the ADA does not specifically state the diseases it covers, the courts have been left to determine disease by disease if it falls under the ADA protection.

If you think an employer has discriminated against you because of your disease, you should seek legal counsel from someone trained in employment laws. Your lawyer will determine if you have a legitimate claim and would then proceed to file one. The Equal Employment Opportunity Commission (EEOC) is the government agency that monitors employers' compliance with laws against employee discrimination.

If you think you are a victim of discrimination, contact the EEOC at (800) 669-4000. The EEOC will look into the matter and if it finds a basis for discrimination, will give you a "right to sue" letter. At this point, you can sue in federal court. If your state has an agency that is authorized to provide relief for discrimination, you must first seek assistance from that agency before you bring charges to the EEOC. You have 180 days after the incident to file charges. If the local agency has stopped processing the charge then you have 300 days after the discriminatory act to bring charges with the EEOC. You can also bring charges in state court at the same time.

You may also use the Equal Pay Act (EPA) to file discrimination charges. Under the EPA, you have up to two years to file charges and you are not required to file charges with the EEOC before filing a private lawsuit.

As shown previously, filing charges against an employer can be very complicated and hence it is highly advisable to seek legal help. Not all lawyers are familiar with employment law, so be sure to find one who has handled these types of cases.

The Rehabilitation Act

This law, passed in 1973, was the first law to protect individuals with disabilities. The law, however, covered only federal agencies and colleges participating in federal student loan programs or receiving federal grants. It also bars discrimination in agencies that receive federal funds and businesses that receive federal contracts. Each federal agency provides its own regulations to govern its own programs. Businesses that receive funds from these agencies have to comply with that agency's regulations on enforcing the Rehabilitation Act.

The Rehabilitation Act was modified after the ADA was passed to provide the same protections to federal employees as the ADA gives to private employees.

Colleges have to make reasonable accommodations for students with disabilities under the Rehabilitation Act. While colleges are expected to make appropriate academic adjustments and reasonable modifications to allow for full participation of students with disabilities, they are not, however, required to provide special educational programs for those with disabilities.

Enforcement under the Rehabilitation Act is the responsibility of each agency with regard to how its regulations are carried out. Individuals may also bring private lawsuits without a "right to sue" letter as with the ADA. For more information about filing complaints under the Rehabilitation Act, contact the civil rights division of the U.S. Department of Justice at (800) 514-0301.

The Family and Medical Leave Act (FMLA)

The FMLA was passed in 1993, and although it is not an antidiscriminatory act, it gives individuals some protections in the workplace as they deal with health issues. The law provides employees up to 12 weeks of unpaid leave to take care of a loved one: a newborn; a newly adopted child; a seriously ill spouse, child, or parent; or one's own serious medical problems. You can take the 12 weeks in any given 12-month period. Your employment is guaranteed; that is, you cannot be fired while you are away. To be covered under the FMLA, a private employer must have at least 50 employees within a 75-mile area. All public employers, federal, state and local, are also covered under the FMLA.

Eligibility

To have your job protected under the FMLA:

- You must have been employed for at least 12 months.
- You must have worked at least 1,250 hours prior to taking the leave.
- If the leave is for a serious medical condition, it must be one that requires in-patient care or the continuous medical care of a healthcare professional.

Other Things to Know about the FMLA

In addition to the information already stated, know the following:

- The employer must maintain health benefits while the employee is on FMLA leave. If the employee does not return to work, the employer may recover the paid premiums during that period.
- An employer must designate a leave as an FMLA leave, usually by a letter to the employee. If this is not done, the employer cannot count the leave toward the employee's FMLA allotment.

- An employee can be required to use all sick days, vacation days, and personal days, before using the FMLA days.
- A leave from work due to an illness can be considered an FMLA leave or a reasonable accommodation under the ADA as described previously. The employer can make that determination. This does not mean, however, that an employee loses FMLA days if an employer uses the reasonable accommodation provision of the ADA.

Enforcement of the FMLA falls under the U.S. Department of Labor (DOL). The Wage and Hour Division, which regulates this law, can be reached at (866) 487-9243.

Employment and Health Insurance

There are two federal laws that affect the ability of employees to maintain their health insurance when they leave their jobs. A lot of workers are afraid to quit their jobs because of fear of losing their health insurance. These laws provide some protection in that regard and hence give employees freedom to move to other jobs without fear of becoming uninsured. The laws are:

- The Consolidated Omnibus Budget Reconciliation Act (COBRA) of 1985
- The Health Insurance Portability and Accountability Act (HIPAA) of 1996

COBRA

COBRA gives employees who belonged to a group health plan in their jobs the opportunity to purchase and maintain the same group health coverage for a period of time, between 18 and 36 months. The dependents of the employee are also eligible for coverage under COBRA. This means that if you had a job where the employer provided insurance to workers through a group plan and you leave that job for any reason— being fired or quitting—the insurance company cannot cut you out of that coverage. This provides you protection while you are looking for a new job or getting different insurance. If the spouse of the employee was covered under the plan, he or she also has this protection, even if they get divorced or the covered spouse dies. Children, either biological or adopted, are also covered. These are some details to be aware of regarding COBRA:

- The law affects only employers with 20 or more employees.
- The insurance has to be a group plan.
- You are responsible for paying the premiums during COBRA coverage.

COBRA, as with all federal laws, sets the basic rights that citizens throughout the country must have. States can add on to these rights and many states have done so with COBRA. Some states, for example, have reduced the number of employees below 20 that an employer can have to be covered under COBRA. Some states have also added a "conversion option" to COBRA, which means that when your COBRA coverage has ended, the insurance company is required to offer you a personal policy now that you are not covered under the employer's group plan anymore. Remember, during COBRA, your coverage was still under the employer's group plan, even though you were the one paying the premium. At the end of COBRA, the insurance company can terminate your coverage completely. The conversion option at least gives you the chance to continue coverage even though the premiums might now be higher. If you have any question about your rights under COBRA, check with your state's insurance department.

HIPAA

HIPAA became effective in 1996 to protect individuals from being refused health insurance. The basic rights that HIPAA provides include limiting the use of preexisting conditions to deny insurance coverage to an individual. Many insurance companies turn down an individual with a preexisting medical condition or do not provide coverage for an illness that existed before the policy was granted. Under HIPAA, if you had group health coverage from your employer and you left that job and are now enrolling in another group plan or individual plan, the new plan cannot refuse to cover you for a medical condition that you already have. In other words, no preexisting medical condition exclusion can be applied to your coverage. To be eligible for HIPAA protection:

- You must have had at least 18 months coverage through a group health plan.
- You are not covered by any other health plan.
- You did not lose coverage because you did not pay your premiums.

- You accepted and used up any conversion option provided by COBRA (see prior section on COBRA) or any other state program.

As with most laws, there are groups or employers who are exempt. These include:

- Employers of fewer than two employees
- State and local government
- Church-sponsored plans
- Self-insured plans

Also, HIPAA does not:

- Require that employers pay for the coverage
- Control the amount of premium charged
- Determine the type of coverage that a group plan should provide
- Require that an employer provide insurance coverage to any or all of its employees

Again as with all federal laws, the states can provide additional benefits beyond what HIPAA provides. If you need to know more about your rights and protections under HIPAA in your state, contact the state's insurance department.

Family Issues

When we get sick or do the things that prevent us from getting sick, we often realize that our state of health affects those related to us either as friends, family, or acquaintances. We should never feel alone in dealing with health issues, and many times the support and encouragement of those close to us are instrumental to our well-being. The costs associated with our relationships when we get sick are largely defined as intangibles; that is, it is very difficult to put a number on them because we really can't define them. How can you measure the pain that arises from a failed marriage because one person was depressed and did not seek help and the other decided the sick person was too emotionally draining and left? As we examine the different aspects of our disease states and how they affect our relationships, it is important to remember that the two most important ways to deal with each stage are communication and planning.

Dealing with the Emotional Cost of Primary Prevention

In primary prevention, the goal is to live a healthy lifestyle to prevent getting sick. The challenge here, in terms of our relationships, is to get the support we need to make the necessary lifestyle changes. If you are the one who initiated the healthy lifestyle, you need the understanding of those around you to help you keep it up. If it is someone else who caused you to change to a healthy lifestyle, you need to understand why the someone is making you do this and seek the person out to help you maintain the change. The key again is communication and the right company. If you are around people who are living healthy lifestyles, it is much easier to change to, and/or maintain, a healthy lifestyle. If you are surrounded by people who are not living healthy lifestyles, it becomes more difficult to live one. For example, it probably would not help if you are trying to quit smoking and are surrounded by people who not only smoke but tell you how difficult it is to stop and that smoking is not that bad. So seek out individuals who are living healthy lifestyles to act as mentors to you.

Communication, too, is key. Any changes you make in your life will most likely affect somebody else. If you decide to take time to engage in a routine exercise program, that could mean spending less time with a loved one who might not appreciate that, especially if he or she doesn't get to see you very much. If you decide to eat more fruits and vegetables and less red meats and fatty foods, this might not sit well with somebody who thinks a meal is not complete without a thick slice of steak. You must, therefore, find a way to convince those affected by the changes you are making why it is important to live the healthy lifestyle you have chosen. You must take into account their feelings and find ways to create the change without damaging your relationship. Maybe you need to institute the changes gradually. Maybe you can solicit the help of an individual whom the person you are trying to convince trusts, such as a minister, an uncle or aunt, or a mutual friend, to help the person see why you are trying to make a change. Communicate, communicate, and communicate some more.

Dealing with the Emotional Cost
of Secondary Prevention

In secondary prevention, the goal is to prevent the disease from becoming complicated and hence more difficult and costly to manage. The key here is to have people who encourage you to do what your healthcare provider told you to do and do it religiously.

You should always involve at least one other trusted individual in every aspect of your healthcare. Do not hide the fact that you have an illness; there is no shame in being ill, and the most important goal is to get well. If you feel ashamed of your illness, then seek the help of someone you trust. There will always be someone to listen to you. If you have to go outside your immediate circle of acquaintances to find that person, call an advocacy group and they will tell you where to go.

When you are dealing with an illness, there are changes in you that those around you might not understand. Family and friends of a person dealing with depression might think the person is just gloomy and difficult to be around. Or a caretaker of an Alzheimer's patient might feel burned out from the stress of caregiving and might resent the behaviors of the patient and the effect of the disease on his or her lifestyle. Family members and acquaintances need to be as educated about the disease as the patient, and also deserve support. The more those around the patient know about the illness that has befallen a loved one, the better they can help and support the patient.

Dealing with Institutional Care Issues
for Patients and Loved Ones

Once a patient moves from home to an institution, be it a hospital or a nursing home, some of the day-to-day care shifts from family and acquaintances to the institution. While there is less burden on direct care, the big issues become the anxiety of knowing the disease is more serious, as well as dealing with the financial burden that institutional care imposes. The key to dealing with these issues is planning. While some diseases that require institutional care do come on suddenly, like strokes or heart attacks, most of the diseases come on gradually and hence we have time to plan for them. As diabetes progresses, as Alzheimer's progresses, as AIDS progresses, we know there may well come a time when the patient might end up in an institution. We should prepare ourselves both emotionally and financially for when that time comes. Nothing can ever take away the pain and suffering of seeing a loved one go into an institution, but planning might lessen the impact.

If the emotional burden is too much, seek professional help. There are also many support groups for those who have a disease as well as for their relatives. Look up these groups in the yellow pages or call the advocacy group for that disease to find out about support groups in your area. If none is available, you might consider starting one. That is how most support groups got started.

In dealing with the financial burden, make sure you or your loved one has adequate health insurance. Explore all avenues available that provide financial support for individuals with that disease or that demographic group. There are many public and private programs that help individuals with specific diseases. The advocacy group for that disease can help you with that information. Talk to a financial planner. With proper financial planning, you might be able to get assistance handling such things as nursing home care or to get public assistance.

Dealing with Death and Dying

When a loved one has a terminal disease, the emotional burden can be truly overwhelming for all involved. The patient goes through what has been described as the five stages of dying: denial, anger, bargaining, depression, and finally acceptance. In the final stage, the person dying is actually at peace with himself or herself and is looking forward to death. For the loved ones, this might be the toughest phase to deal with, as the patient is no longer fighting and they worry that this time could be the last time they see the person alive.

A number of end-of-life issues should be taken care of. These issues fall under what is known as "advanced directives." Advanced directives ensure that when you are dying or when you die, certain actions will be taken on your behalf. Three legal documents will accomplish this: a will, a living will, and a durable power of attorney for healthcare proxy.

A will gives instructions as to what should happen to your estate when you die. A living will gives instructions regarding what should be done for you regarding medical care in the event that you become so sick you cannot functionally take part in the medical decision making. It gives the doctors instructions about how much pain you want to endure. You might instruct that you want to die free of any pain and that in the event of a shutdown in your heart and lung function you do not want to be revived. This is known as a "Do Not Resuscitate" (DNR) order. The directive might also specify what types of procedures you do not want performed and any other measures that you deem might be used to prolong your life. Many studies have shown that the greatest expense to the healthcare system is the cost spent at the end of life, when the patient is dying. For many families, keeping alive a person who has no chance of recovery can be a great financial as well as an emotional burden. Many individuals have DNRs to spare the family from making this choice. However, don't feel compelled to put down a DNR for financial reasons alone even if you feel it will help you avoid pain and you don't feel that it will make a difference in your quality of life. This is a decision that should take into account the emotional impact of those left behind seeing a loved one die.

Because living wills sometime conflict with what doctors are trained to do—to save lives—some states do not recognize them. Ask your attorney, financial planner, or legislator about your state's rules on living wills.

A durable power of attorney for healthcare proxy gives the right to make medical decisions regarding your care to someone you designate in the event that you cannot make those decisions. This can take an emotional toll on the designated individual if he or she is called on to make a life or death decision. Be sure to consult carefully with the person you have chosen and give him or her as many specific directions as you can. All states recognize durable power of attorney for healthcare proxy.

All of these documents are legal documents so consult with a lawyer to get them done. Estate planners advise that all individuals should have these documents as part of a sound estate plan, regardless of their state of health.

PART FOUR

Managing the Cost of Common Chronic Diseases

CHAPTER 9

Alzheimer's Disease

There are about four million individuals in North America with Alzheimer's disease (AD), and each year about 400,000 new cases are diagnosed. It affects mostly older people—those age 65 and older—and the prevalence doubles every five years beyond the age of 65.

Once someone is diagnosed with Alzheimer's, the individual will be expected to live about 8 to 10 years post diagnosis. However, the disease can last for 20 years or longer, meaning that it might take some time before it is diagnosed. Alzheimer's is the most common form of loss of memory and intellectual functioning, or what is clinically referred to as dementia. While we all tend to forget things sometimes, for an individual to be considered to have dementia, he or she must exhibit decline in intellectual and other brain functioning to the point where it affects the conduct of activities that are part of daily living.

What Is Alzheimer's Disease?

Alzheimer's is a progressive and permanent loss of brain functioning that results in memory loss and decline in thinking abilities. It also causes behavior and personality changes. It usually begins gradually and worsens over time, although the rate of decline varies from person to person. While the cause of the disease is not known, it starts as a breakdown in the connections between nerves in the part of the brain that controls memory with formation of abnormal structures called plaques and tangles and leads to the eventual death of the nerve cells. The damage then spreads to the part of the brain that controls language and reasoning.

As the damage progresses, the individual starts by first forgetting recent events or familiar tasks. Eventually, the person starts becoming confused, with accompanying behavior changes and impaired judgment. He or she struggles to find words, finish thoughts, or follow directions, and is unable to take care of himself or herself.

It is important to realize that not all memory and intellectual functioning loss is due to Alzheimer's. There are many conditions or diseases that can result in memory loss, including depression, brain tumor, Huntington's disease, stroke, Parkinson's, and vitamin B_{12} deficiency. The memory loss in these conditions is called non-Alzheimer's type dementia. While the ability to remember decreases with age, cognitive function should remain intact.

Symptoms

As Alzheimer's progresses, it goes through four stages:
- Early stage, or mild AD
- Intermediate stage, or moderate AD
- Severe stage, or severe AD
- End stage

The early stage is characterized by the following symptoms:
- Loss of recent memory
- Inability to learn and retain new information
- Language problems
- Mood swings
- Irritation

In the intermediate stage these symptoms appear:
- Inability to learn new information
- Memory of old events affected
- Assistance needed with daily activities like bathing and eating
- Physically aggressive
- Wandering
- Loss of sense of time and place

In the severe stage, the patient is:
- Unable to walk or perform any activity of normal living

- Faced with both short-term and long-term memory loss
- Unable to eat or swallow
- Very susceptible to bacterial infection
- Increasingly prone to seizure

At the end stage, the patient goes into a coma and dies, usually from an infection.

The Alzheimer's Association has developed a list of 10 symptoms to alert people to the possibility of having Alzheimer's. They are:

1. Memory loss that affects job skills
2. Difficulty performing familiar tasks
3. Problems with language
4. Disorientation in terms of time and place
5. Poor or decreased judgment
6. Problems with abstract thinking
7. Misplacing things
8. Changes in mood or behavior
9. Changes in personality
10. Loss of initiative

Once an individual starts showing signs of these symptoms, a physician should be consulted for complete testing to make a diagnosis.

Prevention

One of the primary goals in managing the cost of Alzheimer's disease is to delay its onset. The hope here is to prevent it all together or at least slow its progression. It has been estimated that if the onset of the disease can be delayed for five years, it would cut in half the number of people with the disease and save the economy as much as $50 billion a year.

A number of compounds are being studied for their potential to delay the onset of Alzheimer's disease, to slow its progression, or prevent it all together. These compounds are:

- Antioxidants
- Anti-inflammatory agents
- Estrogen
- Nerve growth factors

Antioxidants

As part of normal metabolism, the body produces substances known as free radicals. Overproduction or the slowdown in getting rid of free radicals can cause damage to the body. Free radicals also are involved in the aging process and have been shown to play a part in the development of Alzheimer's. The belief, therefore, is that if one can reduce the number of free radicals in the body, one could delay the onset of Alzheimer's. Substances called antioxidants can clean up free radicals. They include:

- Vitamins C and E
- Flavonoids (found in plants like tomatoes)
- Carotenoids (found in plants like carrots)
- Ginkgo biloba
- Melatonin

Vitamin E was shown in a large study to slow down progression of Alzheimer's disease, and is now recommended as part of the treatment for the disease. Several reports have indicated that gingko can improve memory and the government is now supporting several clinical trials to confirm these reports.

Anti-inflammatory Drugs

Inflammation in the brain is present in individuals with Alzheimer's disease. It is not known if the inflammation causes the disease or is present because of the disease. Some studies have shown that anti-inflammatory agents can slow down the formation of plaques in the brain (plaques in the brain are a hallmark of Alzheimer's disease) and the current belief is that anti-inflammatory agents might be able to slow down the disease's progression. A number of studies are using steroids and other types of agents known as nonsteroidal anti-inflammatory agents (NSAIDs), such as Advil or Aleve, to see if they are better than steroids. Some studies are using the newer types of NSAIDs such as Celebrex and Vioxx that cause less stomach irritation to see if they can slow down Alzheimer's. Ask your doctor about the possibility of using NSAIDs.

Estrogen

Estrogen is a hormone that is produced by the ovaries in females. As a female ages, the production of estrogen declines and ceases when she enters menopause. Estrogen has a powerful effect on the area of the brain that deals with memory and the loss of estrogen may worsen the loss of memory. In fact, several studies have shown that estrogen does appear to decrease the risk of Alzheimer's and to improve memory. Estrogen can act both as an antioxidant and an anti-inflammatory agent, and this could explain why it is helpful in delaying the disease. It should be noted, though, that several studies that have used estrogen replacement therapy in women who already had Alzheimer's disease did not show beneficial effects. Estrogen, therefore, might be helpful in slowing down or preventing the onset of the disease, but might not be as useful once the disease is already diagnosed.

Nerve Growth Factor

In Alzheimer's disease certain nerves in the brain that produce a chemical called acetylcholine shrink and eventually die. Certain compounds can prevent nerve cells from dying, and one of the best-known ones is nerve growth factor (NGF). One study has shown that when cells that could produce NGF were implanted in the brain, the shrinkage and loss of those cells that produce acetylcholine were reversed. If this holds true, it might be possible to prevent Alzheimer's disease by implanting NGF-producing cells in the brain. Ongoing studies will provide us with answers.

Managing the Cost

Alzheimer's is one of the most costly diseases to manage—it is the third most expensive disease, behind heart disease and cancer. The annual cost of caring for Alzheimer's patients increases as the severity of the disease increases. As of this writing, for a patient with mild Alzheimer's it is $18,408; for moderate Alzheimer's, $30,096; and for severe Alzheimer's, $36,132 per year.

What makes Alzheimer's so devastating is the fact that it affects the patient in so many ways, both mentally and physically. This in turn severely affects the way the person interacts with others and the way the disease affects those who take care of the patient.

Physically, the Alzheimer's patient becomes very hostile, starts wandering, and is uncooperative. The person also falls more often, loses control of the bladder, and easily develops infections. Someone with Alzheimer's is twice as likely to have hip fractures and has a greater risk of other injuries such as sprains and burns.

Mentally, the patient becomes depressed, anxious, and fearful. The mental disorder tends to spill over to the caregivers of the Alzheimer's patient. Almost 80 percent of caregivers or family members develop depression.

The two main components of costs in Alzheimer's are the medical costs and the cost of long-term care.

Medical Costs

The medical costs are largely from physician visits and medications.

Physician Visits

Since most individuals with Alzheimer's are 65 years and older, they are covered by Medicare. While Medicare will for the most part cover the cost of seeing a physician for evaluation and follow-up care, it is crucial for both the patient and the caregiver to know as much as they can about the disease, what should be expected in an office visit, the types of tests to be administered, what questions to ask the physician, and what to do at home to make the disease more manageable.

The Alzheimer's Association suggests the following questions be asked as part of an ongoing conversation with the physician:

- Are additional tests needed to confirm the diagnosis?
- Can symptoms be treated?
- How much do these treatments cost? Are there side effects? Are the treatments reimbursable?
- What else can be done to alleviate symptoms?
- Are there clinical drug trials being conducted in the area?

During the initial office visit to get a diagnosis for Alzheimer's, the doctor will perform several tests to rule out other reasons for loss of memory and intellectual functioning. Alzheimer's is a disease that is diagnosed by exclusion; that is, everything else has to be ruled out, and if there are no other causes found, then a diagnosis of Alzheimer's is made. The only way to positively identify that the disease was Alzheimer's is when the patient dies and an autopsy is performed.

The physician will perform a thorough exam that will include medical history, a physical exam, and blood counts, and will perform tests to assess the memory, language, and brain skills of the patient. One of the most-used memory tests is known as the Mini–Mental Status Exam. Brain scans can also be done to rule out tumors or strokes. Subject to deductibles and copays, these costs will be handled by Medicare.

Medications

Regular Medicare does not cover prescription drugs. In this section we will discuss ways to deal with the cost of prescription drugs used to treat Alzheimer's disease. It should be noted, however, that because of the complications stated earlier, the Alzheimer's patient is likely to be on several medications to manage the other disorders brought on as a result of Alzheimer's. This includes treatment for depression, agitation, sleeplessness, and infections.

The strategies for dealing with the cost of these medications should be those described in the chapters on managing prescription drug costs (see chapters 4 and 5). Here, we will concentrate on drugs for Alzheimer's disease.

As of this writing, five drugs have been approved for the treatment of Alzheimer's disease:

- Aricept (donepezil)
- Cognex (tacrine)
- Exelon (rivastigmine)
- Hydergine LC (ergoloid mesylate)
- Reminyl (galantamine)

These drugs work by enhancing the production of acetylcholine, the chemical used in brain transmission that is responsible for memory and intellectual function.

The following table shows the frequency of dosage, the prices, and the manufacturers of these drugs.

Drug	Dosage Frequency	Cost of a Month's Starting Dose	Manufacturer*
Aricept	Once a day	$128	Easai/Pfizer
Cognex	4 times a day	$145	First Horizon
Exelon	2 times a day	$125	Novartis
Hydergine LC	3 times a day	$106	Novartis
Reminyl	2 times a day	$120	Janssen

*See appendix B for the phone numbers of the manufacturers.

The choice of which drug to use is based more on side effects and ease of use than on cost. The cost of a month's prescription, as of this writing ranged from $106 to $145. Brand-name substitution (asking for another brand that is less expensive) is usually not an option with Alzheimer's disease. Also, since most of these drugs (at the time of this writing) have no generic equivalents, generic substitution is not an option.

Samples

As stated in chapter 4, it is always a good idea to ask your physician for samples. Samples are a free source of medication and they also help the physician determine if a drug is right for a patient. Physicians, especially primary care physicians such as internists, family practitioners, and general practitioners, as well as specialists like neurologists and psychiatrists, usually have free samples of Alzheimer's medication. As new drugs come out, they are usually heavily sampled; in other words, your doctor will be given a fair amount of the drug to give to his or her patients.

Drug Company Assistance Programs

The makers of Alzheimer's medications are very aware of the fact that most of the patients on these medications are elderly, many of whom do not have prescription drug coverage. These companies, therefore, have generous assistance programs to help individuals who qualify for their assistance. To qualify for these programs, you must not have any insurance that covers prescription drugs and you have to meet their income criteria. To find out the specific qualifications criteria for a particular company, call the company (the numbers are listed in appendix B).

If you don't qualify for the free drug program, ask the company if it offers the newly created discount cards that allow you to get the drug at a much reduced rate.

Pill Cutting

As discussed in chapter 5, while this technique can produce substantial savings on medication costs, it is one that should be done very carefully and sometimes by the pharmacist or physician. The risk of the patient ending up taking the wrong dose is high. The Alzheimer's patient is not in a position to administer this strategy. It is therefore advised that the caregiver of the patient discuss this strategy with the physician and seek the assistance of the pharmacist in using this strategy.

Pill cutting in Alzheimer's produces only short-term savings because most patients eventually end up on the highest dose. Nonetheless, this strategy can be employed in the early treatment phases where the patient is started with the lowest dose.

State Government Assistance Program

All the states that have programs to assist individuals with prescription drug cost designed those programs primarily to address the issue of drug cost for the elderly. Since Alzheimer's is predominantly a disease of the elderly, it is very advisable to explore the assistance programs provided by these states. A lot of Alzheimer's patients also qualify for Medicaid, which in most states covers prescription drugs. See appendix A to find out whether your state has a prescription assistance program.

Other Programs to Assist with Prescriptions

As described in chapter 5, joining a discount pharmacy program can result in substantial savings, especially if the patient is on multiple medications for chronic conditions. Be sure to comparison shop the different programs and compare membership fee and services provided.

Alzheimer's patients who have HMO insurance that covers the cost of their prescription drugs can still realize substantial savings by using the mail order service of the HMO. Ordering by mail is highly recommended because the program will closely monitor the use of the medication and will usually alert the patient when it is time to get a refill. It also saves the patient the need to go to the pharmacy since the drug is delivered to their residence. Again, see chapter 5 for how to use this program.

Disease Management and Participation in Clinical Trials

Early interventions not only can prevent complications that are more costly to manage, but can also delay nursing home care. A nurse or a physician should monitor the patient regularly to identify problems early. This includes checking for infections and signs of malnourishment. Providing palliative care designed for patients with advanced Alzheimer's has been shown to reduce total medical cost almost three times compared to not using palliative care.

Participation in clinical trials is an area to consider for a number of reasons:

- Clinical trials are usually in the forefront of science and are likely to provide interventions that are not yet available to the general public.
- Clinical trials are usually supervised very closely and the patient would most likely receive more care than at home or in a nursing facility.
- Clinical trials are free, and can sometimes pay a small fee to participants.
- Clinical trial participants usually receive thorough medical checkups as part of their evaluation.

That being said, there are a number of issues to be aware of before deciding to participate in a clinical trial:

- Clinical trials are usually designed to test the effectiveness of a drug or procedure. This involves some risk since the drug or procedure might not work and might even cause some unforeseen harm.
- In some trials, not all the participants are given the real medication or procedure. The patient and his or her doctor are usually not aware of who is getting the real medicine until the end of the study.

Long-Term Care: Caregiving

A very significant cost area of managing Alzheimer's is that of caregiving. Every Alzheimer's patient will eventually have to be taken care of either at home by a relative or loved one or in a nursing facility. The impact of taking care of the Alzheimer's patient can be devastating both emotionally and financially.

Alzheimer's patients are usually cared for at first in the home and eventually some move on to nursing homes. Since most of the caring for the Alzheimer's patient occurs at home, families of Alzheimer's patients bear a huge cost, both financially and emotionally.

Alzheimer's caregivers report that they have high levels of stress and are more likely to have the following physical and emotional health problems because of their caregiving:

- They are three times as likely to be depressed.
- One in three uses medication for problems related to caregiving.
- One in eight becomes ill or injured as a result of caregiving.
- They have less time for other family members and sometimes give up vacations and hobbies to take care of the Alzheimer's patient.

The effect of caregiving on businesses is substantial. This cost arises from caregiver absenteeism, loss of productivity, replacing caregivers who leave to care for their loved ones, continuing insurance for workers on leave, fees to temp agencies, and cost of employee assistance programs, as well as the businesses' share of the healthcare cost and research cost for Alzheimer's disease. The cost to businesses is estimated to be almost $35 billion a year.

The single most requested need of caregivers is free time or a break from caregiving. This can be accomplished by using respite care, where someone comes in to take care of the patient for a while and the caregiver takes some time off. The caregiver can also use a daycare facility, where the patient is cared for during the day and the caregiver can have time to do other things. It has been reported that nearly one-third of caregivers who gave up work to become caregivers were able to return to full-time or part-time employment when they started using daycare facilities.

It is advisable to use respite care at the mild and moderate stages of the disease because this can delay nursing home placement.

It has also been shown that when caregivers were given counseling and support services, they were able to take better care of the Alzheimer's patient. This delayed nursing home care by an average of 329 days, compared with caregivers who did not receive counseling and did not participate in a support group. Each month of delay in nursing home care is currently a savings of over $1,800.

Nursing Home Care

Eventually, a lot of Alzheimer's patients end up needing nursing home care. At the present time, Medicare does not pay for long-term care and does not cover home health benefits for Alzheimer's care unless there is a coexisting medical condition that is covered under skilled nursing care.

Medicaid does cover long-term care, but to qualify for this care, the patient must have exhausted enough resources to become poor enough to qualify. When the patient enters a nursing home, his or her income must be turned over to the nursing home and the government then pays out the difference.

While an individual can buy private insurance to cover long-term care, once one is diagnosed with Alzheimer's disease, it is almost impossible to qualify for this, or if one does, the cost may be too high to justify buying it. As most financial planners would advise, everyone should get long-term care insurance when they reach age 55. If, on the other hand, the patient doesn't have such insurance, it is still wise to get it at the earliest stages of diagnosis. In the absence of any policy, and if the patient or family will face crushing medical bills to pay for long-term care, the family should consult a financial planner to see if and how they can qualify for Medicaid.

As these financial arrangements are being handled, it is equally important to take care of some legal issues as well. As discussed in chapter 8, three documents should be obtained: a will, a living will, and a durable power of attorney for healthcare proxy. This should be done as early as possible in the diagnosis. These documents ensure that patients have their wishes acknowledged before they reach a point where they can't make any decisions.

Resources

To learn more about Alzheimer's disease and to find out about local caregiver support groups, call the Alzheimer's Association at (800) 272-3900, or log on to www.alz.org.

To stay abreast of the latest scientific knowledge on Alzheimer's disease, call the Alzheimer's Disease Education and Referral (ADEAR) Center of the National Institute on Aging (NIA) at (800) 438-4380, or log on to www.alzheimers.org.

CHAPTER 10

Arthritis

C urrently, about 43 million Americans have arthritis. Arthritis robs the body of movements that we rely on to do the various activities we have made a part of our lives. It is the leading cause of disability in adults 65 years and older. Arthritis is actually a catchall name that covers about 100 different diseases. What is common to all of them is pain and stiffness in the joints. The causes and treatment of the various forms of arthritis can be very different.

It has been shown that when arthritis is caught early and steps to treat it are initiated before the disease is advanced, joint damage can be significantly reduced and the disability that arthritis causes can be more easily managed. Unfortunately, most people confuse the early symptoms of the disease with something else and wait for a long time before seeking proper treatment.

What Is Arthritis?

In the simplest definition, arthritis is inflammation of the joint. Our body is made up of hundreds of tissues and organs that are connected by joints. The best-known joints are the ones that connect bones. Joints are designed to provide us with flexibility and ease of movement. The ends of the bones are covered by a smooth structure called cartilage and the bones are attached to one another by ligaments. The joints also contain a fluid, called synovial fluid, that acts as a lubricant.

In normal operations, the ligaments allow bones to move with each other in the joints. With synovial fluid providing the lubrication, the movements are painless. In arthritis, the joint starts becoming worn down or inflamed. The bones might start touching each other, the synovial fluid might increase in volume and cause swelling, the ligaments might snap, or other structures in the joint might become damaged. As this occurs, normal movement of the joint becomes painful and the joint is now termed arthritic.

Symptoms

The different types of arthritis have different symptoms and each one has its own unique feature. There are, however, certain symptoms that can lead to a diagnosis of arthritis:

- Swelling in one or more joints
- Stiffness around the joints that lasts for at least one hour in the early morning
- Constant or recurring pain or tenderness in a joint
- Difficulty using or moving a joint normally
- Warmth and redness in a joint

Some of these symptoms occur in other diseases; for example, individuals with Parkinson's disease experience stiffness. Cardiovascular disease might lead to swellings called edema. If you start experiencing any of the symptoms listed above, it is important to see your doctor to get the right diagnosis so that appropriate treatment can be initiated.

Types

There are more than 100 types of arthritis. The two most common types are osteoarthritis and rheumatoid arthritis.

Osteoarthritis

Osteoarthritis (OA) is the most common form of arthritis, affecting about 21 million adults in the United States. It results when the cartilage that protects the ends of the bones becomes inflamed. The cartilage can become completely worn out to the point of actual bone-to-bone contact. Pointy bulges of bone then start appearing on the ends of the bones.

The wearing down and decay of the cartilage is thought to arise from the constant and daily mechanical use of the joints. As one gets older the chances of developing osteoarthritis increases. Some people, however, never develop OA no matter how old they get. Certain risk factors, such as being overweight, increase the chances of getting OA.

Osteoarthritis develops gradually, usually involving one or more joints. The telltale signs are:

- Pain that is worsened by exercise and relieved by rest
- Morning stiffness that follows inactivity and lasts less than 30 minutes and is improved by activity

The disability brought about by OA is usually felt when it attacks the big bones. The most affected areas are the spine and weight-bearing bones like the hips and knees.

Rheumatoid Arthritis

Rheumatoid arthritis (RA) is the second most common form of arthritis, affecting about 2 million people. It occurs two to three times more often in women than in men, hence it is felt that hormones or some other male-female difference might play a role in its development. It can occur at any age but usually is initially diagnosed in those between 25 and 50 years old. There may also be a genetic link that predisposes one to develop RA if there is a family history of RA.

In RA, the body starts attacking itself, and the top lining of the cartilage becomes inflamed and swollen. Rheumatoid arthritis usually attacks joints of the extremities. The symptoms of RA are:

- Pain in the joints of the wrists, fingers, and toes
- Swellings of symmetrical joints (occurring equally on both sides of the body)
- Stiffness that lasts over 30 minutes upon arising (morning stiffness) or after prolonged inactivity

The symptoms usually develop slowly but may be abrupt, with many joints being affected at the same time.

Ankylosing Spondylitis

This is one of the few types of arthritis that is more common in men than in women. It affects primarily the spine, causing back pain. It tends to affect individuals in late adolescence or early adulthood.

Fibromyalgia

This is characterized by pain and stiffness of muscles and tissues that support and move bones and joints. The symptoms are worsened by environmental factors such as a job, as well as stress, depression, and anxiety. Patients may experience fatigue and sleep disturbance.

Gout

Gout is caused when needlelike crystals of a substance called uric acid accumulate in the joints. The body produces uric acid as a waste product, and the uric acid is sent out through the urine. People with gout produce an excess amount of uric acid that turns to crystals and accumulates in tendons, ligaments, and cartilage of joints, causing pain. The big toe is the area most affected.

Lupus

Clinically known as systemic lupus erythematosus (SLE), lupus is like rheumatoid arthritis in that the body attacks itself. It occurs 90 percent of the time in women. It is an inflammation of what are known as connective tissues, in the joints, skin, kidneys, heart, lungs, blood vessels, and brain.

Prevention

In arthritis, much of the emphasis is on secondary prevention, in that once you have been diagnosed with arthritis, there are many things that can be done to limit its effects and give the patient as normal a life as is possible. The reason primary prevention is difficult is because arthritis is usually caused by mechanical wear and tear that comes from having used a joint over a long period of time or from an autoimmune disease where the body begins attacking itself. In all of these cases, there isn't much that can be done to prevent it. You can't stop using your joints as you get older in life, and at the present time, we do not have the technology to effectively control the genes that turn on the body to attack itself.

Nevertheless, a healthy lifestyle (see chapter 2) can go long way to actually delay the onset of arthritis and in a few individuals may even prevent it. Exercise and proper nutrition can be very helpful in holding some arthritis at bay. Exercise keeps the joints flexible and encourages adequate lubrication. Not only does proper nutrition provide the body with the ingredients needed to produce the structures that create good joints, but weight management ensures that the joints are not bearing more than they can handle. An obese person puts a tremendous burden on weight-bearing joints, which leads to increased wear and tear and hence increases the chances of osteoarthritis.

Secondary prevention comes essentially from things that are done to treat arthritis. The goal in arthritis therapy is to reduce the pain, increase joint flexibility, and reduce further damage. The different approaches include:

- Rest and relaxation
- Exercises
- Hot and cold therapy
- Assistive devices
- Medications
- Surgery

Rest and Relaxation

It is important to rest and relax, especially with the types of arthritis that cause fatigue, such as rheumatoid arthritis. Rest gives the body time to recoup and this reduces the pain. It is important to note, however, that too much rest can result in joint stiffness, so alternate constantly between rest and activity. A form of relaxation known as progressive relaxation, whereby the patient tightens a muscle and then slowly releases the tension, has been shown to reduce pain.

Exercise

Exercise can reduce pain and stiffness, and increase muscle strength and endurance. It can also help in weight reduction, which is good for weight-bearing joints. Three types of exercises should be part of an exercise program in aiding an arthritic patient:

- Range-of-motion exercises, designed to increase flexibility and maintain joint movement
- Strengthening exercises for muscles
- Aerobic exercises to improve cardiovascular fitness, increase endurance, and reduce inflammation

A popular form of exercise is hydrotherapy, in which the patient exercises in a large pool of warm water. Exercising in water takes some weight off the joints and the warmth helps to increase flexibility.

Hot and Cold Therapies

Heat increases blood flow, tolerance for pain, and flexibility. Heat can be applied through various methods, including paraffin wax, ultrasound, microwave, or steam. Cold numbs the nerves, reducing pain, and also reduces inflammation and muscle spasms.

Cold therapy can be achieved through soaking in cold water, and using ice packs, sprays, or ointments that cool the skin.

Assistive Devices

As arthritis progresses, the joints become weaker and help is needed to not only reduce the workload on the joint, but also to support the joint. This is accomplished by using various devices such as splints and braces. An arthritic patient can also use a cane when walking to take some load off the joints. Shoe inserts can ease the pain of arthritis in the foot and knee.

Medications

Medications are used to decrease the pain and inflammation of the joints. We will discuss them in the cost section that follows. Medications do not cure arthritis, except in the case where the arthritis was caused by an infection, such as in Lyme disease. Medications, however, provide valuable relief from pain and some of them can actually decrease the inflammation and reduce stiffness.

Surgery

The damage to the joint can be so severe that the joint must be surgically repaired or even replaced. Some surgeries are minor, done to repair damaged ligaments, and some are major, like replacing a hip or fusing bones in a joint.

Managing the Cost

In 1992 (the last year for which numbers are available), the cost of managing arthritis was estimated at about $65 billion. Of this, $15 billion was from direct costs and $50 billion from indirect costs. Direct costs are those incurred from treating the disease, while indirect costs come from wages lost from jobs and implied lost wages from reduced homemaking activities. Another cost, called intangible cost, comes from social disability and its impact on relationships.

Direct Costs

The main components of the direct costs in managing arthritis are:

- Physician services
- Medications
- Exercise programs
- Assistive devices
- Institutional care

Physician Services

Unlike a silent disease like high blood pressure, with arthritis you know that something is wrong. When you start experiencing the symptoms listed previously and they do not go away after a while, you should see a doctor to determine what is wrong. The physician will diagnose arthritis based on the history and physical examination of the patient. The physical examination involves checking for joint motion, increased heat in the joint, tenderness, and degree of swelling. Laboratory and X-ray measurements complement what the physician already suspects.

The cost of physician visits in arthritis comes mostly from frequent visits to the physician and having him or her evaluate the effectiveness of the therapy. For the most part, there aren't a lot of procedures to be done except when the disease has progressed to the point where intervention in the joint is needed. Physician visits are easily handled by copays for those with managed care policies. As with all managed care contracts, be sure you closely follow the plan's procedure in terms of seeing your primary care physician and staying within the network of physicians. If you have to see a specialist, usually a rheumatologist (someone who specializes in diseases of the joints) or an orthopedic surgeon, get the proper referrals. This will prevent you from having to pay for the visits and any procedures from out of your pocket. If you have indemnity insurance, then you will pay your share of the cost, as stated in your policy.

If You Don't Have Insurance

If you do not have insurance, remember that the cost of physician visits, is largely driven by how often you visit the physician and whether the physician is a specialist. You can reduce the number of times you visit a physician by getting as much as you can from every visit you make. This means making sure you thoroughly understand what your disease is, how it is being treated, and what you can do at home to make sure the disease is properly managed. If you are not sure, call your doctor and ask.

Stick with primary care physicians (PCPs) rather than specialists for as long as you can. Most arthritis cases can be managed by PCPs and you might never need a specialist, who is much more expensive. If your PCP determines that you do need a specialist, get a list of names and call around for both reputation and price. Prices for services do vary among physicians.

In chapter 6, we discussed different ways to obtain physician services when you do not have health insurance. These included using facilities at school and at work, neighborhood clinics, and teaching hospitals. One source of physician services, the emergency room, is usually not an option in arthritis because arthritis is usually not considered an emergency. So if you visit the emergency room, you will not get the protection of the law that requires emergency rooms to provide services to patients in an emergency even if they cannot pay for it.

Medications

All the drugs used in managing arthritis can be categorized as:

- Analgesics, used to reduce pain
- Anti-inflammatory, to reduce the inflammation
- Disease-modifying, where the drugs can actually attack the disease itself instead of just providing symptomatic relief.

Many analgesics and anti-inflammatory drugs are available over the counter. Drugs such as Advil, aspirin, Motrin, and Tylenol will reduce pain. Advil, aspirin, and Motrin also reduce inflammation and belong to a class of drugs known as nonsteroidal anti-inflammatory drugs (NSAIDs). Most prescription arthritis drugs fall in this category. Steroids can also be used to reduce inflammation.

Disease-modifying antiarthritic (DMA) drugs are usually used in rheumatoid arthritis. These drugs take much longer to start showing effects, sometimes as long as six months. They work this slowly because they are actually causing changes in the body's immune system.

The following table lists the prescription drugs used to manage arthritis and their manufacturers.

Class	Brand Names	Cost of a Month's Starting Dose	Manufacturer*
Nonsteroidal anti-inflammatory drugs (NSAIDs)	Anaprox DS	$43	Roche
	Cataflam	$128	Novartis
	Celebrex	$86	Pharmacia/Pfizer
	Daypro	$100	Pharmacia
	Dolobid	$64	Merck
	Feldene	$107	Pfizer
	Lodine XL	$49	Wyeth
	Naprelan	$76	Elan
	Naprosyn	$47	Roche
	Orudis	$114	Wyeth
	Oruvail	$89	Wyeth
	Vioxx	$78	Merck
	Voltaren	$73	Novartis
Steroids	Decadron	$28	Merck
	Deltasone	$5	Pharmacia
	Medrol	$25	Pharmacia
	Pediapred	$30	Celltech
	Prelone	$28	Muro
Antirheumatics	Arava	$226	Aventis
	Enbrel	$1,028	Wyeth
	Imuran	$44	Promethus
	Neoral	$49	Novartis
	Plaquenil	$88	Sanofi-Synthelabo
	Rheumatrex	$57	Lederle
	Ridaura	$136	Prometheus

*See appendix B for the phone numbers of the manufacturers.

As you can see, there are different classes of drugs and within each class there are different drugs. The costs of these drugs can range from as low as $5 to as high as $1,100 for a month's supply. While these prices might not be the ones in your neighborhood, the differences in cost within the drugs will probably be the same. So, if your physician determines that you need a class of drugs, you can request a less expensive one to start with. Also, remember that there are over-the-counter drugs for NSAIDs, like aspirin, Motrin, Advil, and Aleve. Ask your doctor about these drugs before using a prescription NSAID. The one drawback of many NSAIDs is that they can cause bleeding of the stomach, which can be very severe, although some NSAIDs are thought to cause less stomach bleeding. Discuss your particular situation with your doctor and let your own experience be your guide.

Brand-Name Substitution

The exchange of one drug in a class for another in the same class to treat a disease is known as brand-name or therapeutic substitution. This technique is used frequently in arthritis therapy because many patients become dissatisfied with their medication, either because of side effects or because they believe it is not effective enough in controlling their pain. There are many choices of drugs, and price can become a factor, especially if you are paying for it. Talk to your doctor about this option.

Generic Substitution

The following brand-name drugs are available in generic forms. If your doctor decides that one of these might be helpful to manage your arthritis, you should get the generic unless, and this is rare, you have a problem or reaction to the generic. Remember, generics are always cheaper than the brand-name drug and yet are made up of the same medicine.

Brand Name	Generic Name
Anaprox DS	Naproxen
Cataflam	Diclofenac
Decadron	Dexamethasone
Deltasone	Prednisone
Dolobid	Diflunisal
Feldene	Piroxicam
Lodine	Etodolac
Medrol	Methyprednisolone
Naprelan	Naproxen
Naprosyn	Naproxen

Brand Name	Generic Name
Neoral	Cyclosporine
Orudis	Ketoprofen
Oruvail	Ketoprofen
Plaquenil	Hydroxychloroquine
Prelone	Prednisolone
Rheumatrex	Methotrexate
Riduara	Aurofin
Voltaren-XR	Diclofenac

Drug Assistance Programs

Every major drug manufacturer has a program to give away free medicine to those with low incomes who have no prescription drug coverage. As stated in chapter 5, these criteria are not written in stone. Even if you think you have a high income, if your medication bill is a significant expense and creates a financial burden, you might qualify. If you have insurance but the insurance doesn't cover prescription drugs (for example, Medicare) or your insurance covers prescription drugs but you are prescribed a medication that your plan doesn't cover, you still might qualify. (See appendix B for the phone numbers of the manufacturers.) If you have a prescription for any of these products, call the number and find out if you qualify for free medications. If you need help with the paperwork, call one of the companies listed in chapter 5 for assistance. If a manufacturer is not listed, then that manufacturer did not offer a prescription assistance program at the time of this writing.

Other Medication Strategies

There are other things you can do to reduce your drug costs. These include:

- Mail order
- State programs
- Samples
- Discount pharmacy programs
- Using the Internet
- Pill cutting
- Importing medication
- Discount drug company programs

Chapters 4 and 5 describe in detail how to use these programs. The more programs you use, the bigger the savings you will realize.

Exercise Programs

Your doctor will work with you to design an exercise program that will help you with your arthritis. You might have to do these exercises on your own at home or in a gym, or you might be referred to a rehabilitation facility that specializes in these programs. Since this is part of your arthritis therapy, your insurance will most probably cover the services. In terms of any exercise equipment that you might buy, check with your insurance plan to determine if they will reimburse you for it.

If your insurance doesn't cover your exercise programs and/or equipment or if you do not have insurance, as long as your physician prescribed the program, your expense could be a tax-deductible item. Check with a tax adviser, because there are limitations on how much you can deduct.

Assistive Devices

As with an exercise program, assistive devices to help you manage your arthritis may be covered by your insurance plan. They might also qualify as tax deductions. Remember, though, that even if an item is tax-deductible it doesn't mean it won't cost you money. It simply means that the government will give you back part of the expenses. So be smart when you shop for these items. Call around and compare prices. Contact the Arthritis Foundation for advice on what type of equipment to get and on how much you should expect to pay. Their number is listed at the end of this chapter.

Institutional Care

Surgery to repair the damage caused by arthritis is one of the most common reason for hospitalizations. Some procedures can be done on an outpatient basis and the patient gets to go home the same day. Some require longer hospital stays.

The seven main types of surgery to repair arthritic damage are:

- Arthrodesis, where bones are fused together
- Arthroscopy, where a thin tube is used to remove loose growth in the joint

- Arthroplasty, where the joint is rebuilt
- Osteotomy, where bone damage is corrected by cutting the bone
- Resection, removal of all or part of a bone
- Synovectomy, removal of the lining of the top layer of the bone
- Total joint replacement, where artificial structures are used to replace severely damaged joints

The cost of these procedures varies in relation to their complexity. Any time a hospital stay accompanies a procedure, the costs increase. As you recall from chapter 7, the hospital has a "hotel" function and a "medical" function. The procedures go under the medical function and they can be expensive. If you have insurance, remember to check with your plan about what they will or will not cover. Pay strict attention to using network, as opposed to nonnetwork, hospitals. Nonnetwork hospitals will cost you more and sometimes might not be covered.

Also, inquire about rehabilitation, which is almost always required after surgery to correct damage from arthritis. Find out what your plan covers. There may be physical therapy facilities that are in your plan's network. Make use of them.

If You Do Not Have Insurance

If you do not have insurance, follow the guidelines outlined in chapter 7 for getting help with hospital costs. As a reminder, public hospitals are the least expensive, and specialty hospitals the most. If at all possible, avoid hospitals that specialize in joint diseases. While they might have more expertise, they are usually very expensive. The surgeries for joint damage can be done very effectively in many community hospitals.

Indirect Costs

The indirect costs come from lost productivity, either at the job or at home. RA is particularly devastating because it can affect younger individuals and once this happens, their ability to work can become seriously endangered. In one study, it was shown that patients who were diagnosed with RA lost 50 percent of their earning capacity within nine years of the disease onset.

Individuals with arthritis are protected under the Americans with Disability Act (ADA; see chapter 8). This law gives disabled individuals protection in the workplace and requires that employers make reasonable accommodations so individuals can carry out the essential functions of their jobs. You cannot be discriminated against because of your arthritis. You should enjoy all the rights and benefits that other workers enjoy.

The ADA protections, however, do not mean that the employer can relax the job requirements to accommodate the disabled individual. What this means, therefore, is that people with arthritis should engage in jobs that allow them to produce as well as nonarthritic individuals. Ask your employer to provide you with the assistance you need to accomplish your job.

Other laws protect those with a disease so they can manage it without fear of losing their jobs. The Family Medical Leave Act, described in chapter 8, is one of those laws. It gives individuals up to 12 weeks of unpaid leave to deal with medical issues, either for themselves or a relative. They cannot be fired because they took such time off.

Intangible Costs

Arthritis can be devastating to one's quality of life, as well as one's relationships. Nearly every aspect of one's life can be affected. Simple activities of daily living, like eating, grooming, and household chores, become difficult, and the physical pain can lead to psychological pain, when one starts feeling helpless and relies more on others. The loss of a hobby because of arthritis is a one-two punch. First you suffer from the physical pain and now you are losing something that used to bring you pleasure.

It has been observed that children with arthritis suffer psychologically from low self-esteem, depression, and concern for their body image.

Relationships can be severely tested when arthritis is present. Sexual difficulties are common because of pain, reduced flexibility, fatigue, and the depression that usually accompanies arthritis.

Dealing with these issues requires communication with loved ones, as well as the counsel of mental health professionals if the psychological pain becomes an issue. Educating those around the patient and confronting the issue can go a long way toward minimizing the problem. It is always important to remember that the disease is no one's fault and that emotional support can truly be of benefit.

Complementary and Alternative Therapy

Arthritis is one of those diseases that creates such discomfort that people go to great lengths to seek relief. Many individuals therefore try a host of nonconventional therapies in the hope of finding relief. A host of complementary and alternative therapies have been used to provide pain relief, including:

- *Acupuncture.* Acupuncture uses needles, inserted in specific points in the skin, to stimulate specific areas. The goal is to restore the proper balance of vital energy or qi (pronounced chi). The yin and the yang of life's forces are expected to be brought back into equilibrium and by so doing, restore the body to good health. Originating in China, acupuncture is one of the oldest known medical practices. It has been used for centuries to deal with a range of conditions, from addiction to pain to emotional ailments.
- *Massage.* In massage therapy, the manipulations are gentle. Various types of massage techniques are available, with each emphasizing a particular body part or manipulation. Massages provide pain relief and reduce levels of stress.
- *Chiropractic.* The chiropractor manipulates the spine to align it a certain way. Chiropractors believe that pain and many diseases come about because the spine is not aligned properly. Pain reduction often occurs with proper alignment of the spine.

In terms of over-the-counter supplements, two have been shown to provide relief, especially in osteoarthritis, and hence are widely used. They are chondroitin and glucosamine. Both of these substances occur naturally in the body. Chondroitin helps to make cartilage more elastic, and glucosamine plays a role in cartilage formation and repair. A large study in Australia indicated that users of chondroitin showed a 60 percent improvement in pain compared to only 20 percent improvement in those not using chondroitin. Other studies have shown improvement in pain with chondroitin usage. Studies with glucosamine have also yielded positive results in patients with osteoarthritis.

Because of these positive results, the government is now sponsoring a massive study to put a definite stamp on these products. The results will be out in 2004. As with the use of any complementary therapy, be sure to let your doctor know if you are taking any of these supplements.

Resources

American Academy of
Orthopedic Surgeons
(800) 824-2663
www.aaos.org

American Chronic Pain
Association
(916) 632-0922
www.theacpa.org

American College of
Rheumatology
(404) 633-3777
www.rheumatology.org

American Pain Society
(847) 375-4715
www.ampainsoc.org

American Physical Therapy
Association
(800) 999-2782
www.apta.org

Arthritis Foundation
(800) 283-7800
www.arthritis.org

National Institute of Arthritis and
Musculoskeletal and Skin
Diseases
(877) 226-4267
www.niams.nih.org

CHAPTER 11

Asthma

Asthma is the leading cause of hospitalizations and school absenteeism for children in the United States. It is one of the most common chronic diseases, affecting about 15 million people. Of that number, 5 million are children. The prevalence of asthma has been increasing steadily since 1980, and while this increase is true for all ages and races and both sexes, the prevalence is higher in children, females, and African Americans. In children, more males than females are affected. Asthma tends to run in families, so individuals with siblings or parents with asthma are more likely to develop the disease.

The rate of increase in asthma and its effect on the health of those involved is causing alarm in the medical community. In 1995, for example, asthma was responsible for 1.5 million hospital emergency visits and about 500,000 hospitalizations. Almost 6,000 people died from asthma attacks. Three times more blacks than whites die from having asthma.

What Is Asthma?

As we breathe, the air moves down a large pipe called the trachea to two smaller pipes called bronchi. The bronchi go into our two lungs. Inside the lungs, the bronchi divide into smaller pipes called bronchioles, which end in small sacs called alveoli. It is in the alveoli that oxygen enters our blood and carbon dioxide leaves our blood.

Muscles that control the flow of air surround all the tubes that bring air into our lungs. In normal conditions, these muscles are relaxed and they let air move freely in and out of our lungs. In an asthma attack, these muscles contract, the tubes become obstructed, and air cannot move freely. The body starts to starve for oxygen and there is a buildup of carbon dioxide.

A number of factors have been identified as agents that can start an asthma attack, including:

- Exercise
- Dust mites
- Mold
- Pollen
- Cockroach waste
- Viruses

Asthmatics react differently to these different factors. In every case, however, the trigger results in obstruction of the airway. Airways become obstructed in three ways:

- Tightening of the muscles surrounding the airways
- Inflammation of the airway lining
- Increased secretion of mucus in the airway

Tightening of the Muscles Surrounding the Airways

When we breathe, we take in substances like smoke, dust, and pollen. In most people, these substances are expelled harmlessly out of the body without us even being aware of having inhaled them. In asthmatics, for one reason or another, the muscles that surround the airways react violently to these triggers and go into a state of contraction. This is known as bronchospasm because of the twitching or spasm that the tubes start experiencing. As this occurs, the individual has a hard time breathing.

Inflammation of the Airway Lining

For one reason or another, the lining of the airways can become inflamed, usually by the same triggers that can cause the airway muscles to become spastic. When the airway lining becomes inflamed, it takes in fluid. It is also invaded by white blood cells. As this occurs it becomes swollen and obstructs the flow of air. The inflammation of the airway lining can also cause the muscles surrounding the airways to start contracting, creating a double-jeopardy situation.

Increased Secretion of Mucus in the Airway

The airway lining is normally covered by a thin layer of mucus. The mucus not only lubricates the airways but also acts as a trap to catch foreign objects like pollen and dust to get rid of them. When the airways become inflamed, the triggers cause the body to produce too much mucus in an attempt to get rid of them. As this happens, the overproduction of the mucus itself becomes a source of obstruction as it starts to clog the airways.

Symptoms

There are signs that alert us that someone might be experiencing an asthma attack. If any of the following symptoms are being experienced, the individual should be evaluated for an asthma attack:

- Coughing
- Wheezing (a whistling noise when breathing)
- Chest tightness (feeling like someone is sitting on or squeezing the chest)
- Shortness of breath

Generally, the attack begins with wheezing and coughing, which could be brief and mild. On other occasions, this can progress, sometimes rapidly, to tightness in the chest and respiratory distress, where the patient is struggling to take in air. The coughing during acute attacks sounds "tight" and usually does not produce mucus. As the attack subsides, mucus production starts to increase. In some children, an asthma attack starts as an itch over the chest or the front part of the neck. Also, a dry cough at night and during exercise could be warning signs.

In a severe asthma attack, the patient experiences fatigue and may be unable to speak more than a few words without stopping for breath. Breathing becomes shallow and the patient becomes confused. An asthma attack can last from a few minutes to several days.

Classification

Asthma is classified into four groups based on the severity and frequency of the attack. The classification also determines the extent and course of therapy. The following table spells out the various classes of asthma attacks.

Class	Days with Symptoms	Nights with Symptoms
Mild intermittent	Less than 2 per week	Less than 2 per month
Mild persistent	Between 3 and 6 per week	Between 3 and 4 per month
Moderate persistent	Daily	Greater than 5 per month
Severe persistent	Continual	Frequent

Your doctor will perform clinical tests to evaluate your lung function in order to determine which group you fit into and hence what course of therapy to pursue.

Complications

The complications arising from acute and chronic asthma attack can range from mild discomfort to death.

In acute attacks, the complications arise in essence from collapse of the lung as the airways become tightened and mucus builds up. There is a real struggle to get air in through the closed airways or to get oxygen through all the fluid.

In chronic attacks, especially when the asthma started in childhood and has persisted for a long period of time, the individual might develop a "squared off" chest where, because of the prolonged breathing difficulties, the chest appears to be in a permanent state of inflation. The breastbone becomes bowed, instead of straightened, and the diaphragm (the muscle separating the chest from the stomach), becomes flatter instead of domed.

The ultimate complication in an asthma attack is the cutoff of airflow into the lungs, resulting in the body being starved of oxygen and preventing the release of carbon dioxide. As this state persists, the individual becomes tired, distressed, and confused, and in the absence of any help will die.

Prevention

Educational efforts aimed at preventing asthma attacks have been shown to reduce significantly the cost of managing asthma. Primary prevention in asthma is designed to prevent an asthma attack from starting in the first place. Secondary prevention is designed to reduce the severity of an asthma attack. Right now, we will focus on primary prevention. Later in the chapter, in the section on medications, we will discuss secondary prevention.

It is important to understand that asthma is a chronic disease that can be effectively managed but cannot be cured. Once someone has asthma, his or her airways will always be sensitive and hence the person is always at risk for an asthma attack.

The National Heart, Lung, and Blood Institute has developed the following guide to help asthmatics reduce their contact with known triggers.

Animal Dander

- Keep furred or feathered pets out of your home. If you can't keep the pet outdoors, keep the pet out of your bedroom and keep the bedroom door closed.
- Cover the air vents in your bedroom with heavy material to filter the air.
- Remove carpets and furniture covered with cloth from your home. If that is not possible, keep the pet out of the rooms where these types of furniture are.

Cockroach Waste

- Keep all food out of your bedroom.
- Keep food and garbage in closed containers (never leave food out).
- Use traps, poison baits, powders, gels, or paste (e.g., boric acid).
- If a spray is used to kill roaches, stay out of the room until the odor goes away.

Dust Mites

- Encase your mattress in a special dust-proof cover.
- Encase your pillow in a special dust-proof cover or wash the pillow each week in hot water. Water must be hotter than 130°F to kill the mites.
- Wash the sheets and blankets on your bed each week in hot water.

Exercise, Sports, Work, or Play

- You should be able to be active without symptoms. See your doctor if you have asthma when you are active, such as when you exercise, do sports, play, or work hard.
- Ask your doctor about taking medicine before you exercise to prevent symptoms.
- Warm up for about 6 to 10 minutes before you exercise.
- Try not to work or play hard outside when the air pollution or pollen levels (if you are allergic to pollen) are high.

Indoor Mold

- Fix leaky faucets, pipes, or other sources of water.
- Clean moldy surfaces with a cleaner that has bleach in it.

Pollen and Outdoor Mold

- Try to keep your windows closed.
- If possible, stay indoors with windows closed during the midday and afternoon, when pollen and some mold spore counts are highest.
- Ask your doctor whether you need to take or increase anti-inflammatory medicine before the allergy season starts.

Smoke, Strong Odors, and Sprays

- If possible, do not use a wood-burning stove, kerosene heater, or fireplace.
- Try to stay away from strong odors and sprays, such as perfume, talcum powder, hair spray, and paints.

Tobacco Smoke

- If you smoke, ask your doctor for ways to help you quit. Ask family members to quit smoking too.

- Do not allow smoking in your home or around you.
- Be sure no one smokes at your child's daycare center.

Vacuum Cleaning
- Try to get someone else to vacuum for you once or twice a week, if you can. Stay out of rooms while they are being vacuumed and for a short while afterward.
- If you must vacuum, use a dust mask, a double-layered or micro-filter vacuum cleaner bag, or a vacuum cleaner with a HEPA filter.

Other Things You Should Do
- Reduce indoor humidity to less than 50 percent. Dehumidifiers or central air conditioners can do this.
- Try not to sleep or lie on cloth-covered cushions or furniture.
- Remove carpets from your bedroom and those laid on concrete, if you can.
- Keep stuffed toys out of the bed or wash the toys weekly in hot water.
- Get a flu shot.
- Do not drink beer or wine or eat shrimp, dried fruit, or processed potatoes if they cause asthma symptoms.
- Cover your nose and mouth with a scarf on cold or windy days.
- Tell your doctor about all the medicines you take, including cold medicines, aspirin, and even eyedrops.

Managing the Cost

In 1998, the cost of managing asthma was estimated at $11.3 billion dollars. The direct costs were $7.5 billion, with the rest attributed to indirect costs.

Direct Costs

The direct costs came from doctor's visits, medications, and hospitalizations. The largest share of direct cost was from hospitalizations, which accounted for 35 percent of the total cost of managing asthma.

The Asthma and Allergy Foundation of America estimated that in 1994, expenditures on medications were experiencing explosive growth, with prescriptions for asthma rising 103.2 percent since 1985. Medications are now becoming the most expensive component of the direct cost of asthma management.

Physician Visits

When an individual starts exhibiting the signs and symptoms of an asthma attack and visits a doctor, the goal is to determine if the person is actually asthmatic and, if so, what degree of lung function is affected. A thorough history will be taken to rule out other lung diseases. The single most important test is a pulmonary function test, whereby the doctor determines the amount and speed of air going into and out of the lungs. A person who has asthma will have normal lung functions when they are not having an attack. This is how the doctor will distinguish asthma from other chronic obstructive lung diseases like emphysema. Sometimes your primary care physician will refer you to a pulmonologist, or lung doctor, who can make a better assessment of your lung function. You might also be sent to an allergist, who might be able to determine what triggers your asthma attack.

If asthma is diagnosed, the physician will design a treatment goal to achieve the following:

- No symptoms or reduce the degree of symptoms
- Sleeping through the night without asthma symptoms
- No time off from school or work due to asthma
- Full participation in physical activities
- No emergency room visits or stays in the hospital
- Little or no side effects from asthma medication

Education about the disease is key in asthma management. Your physician will help you understand what can trigger asthma attacks and how to avoid them. In fact, he or she will probably test you to determine if they can find what triggers your asthma. If they find the trigger, you will be told to avoid situations that expose you to that trigger.

Your doctor will also show you how to take your medicine. Most acute attacks are treated by the use of inhalers. So it is important to know how to use one correctly. Your doctor will show you what to do in an acute attack and what to do even when you do not have attacks.

Nearly all insurance companies have developed extensive asthma management programs. Insurance companies will not only cover the cost of physician visits but will provide other resources, especially for children, to help in the management of asthma. Insurance companies will also pay for the cost of visiting a specialist. Just be sure to follow the procedure for seeing a specialist. This might mean getting a referral from your primary care physician.

If You Do Not Have Insurance

If you do not have insurance, make use of the services described in chapter 6 for obtaining physician services. Since asthma affects so many children, the use of school health facilities represents a source of medical care. Individuals with health facilities at their work site should also look at using them. A lot of asthmatics end up in the emergency room because of an asthma attack. However, it is essential to have follow-up care after leaving the hospital. If you can't afford a private doctor, use a neighborhood clinic that receives federal funds. These clinics are expected to care for the uninsured or underinsured and they can work out payment plans with you.

Medications

Two types of medications are used to combat asthma: the fast-acting medications given when an attack is occurring, and the long-acting medications given to prevent attacks.

Fast-Acting Medications for Quick Relief

Class	Brand Names	Cost of a Month's Starting Dose	Manufacturer*
Inhaled beta agonists	Alupent	$30	Boehringer Ingelheim
	Brethaire	$30	Bristol-Myers Squibb
	Maxaire	$47	3M
	Proventil	$30	Schering
	Ventolin	$32	GlaxoSmithKline

Long-Acting Medications for Secondary Prevention

Class	Brand Name	Cost of a Month's Starting Dose	Manufacturer*
Long-acting inhaled beta agonists	Serevent	$70	GlaxoSmithKline
Inhaled steroids	Aerobid	$120	Forest
	Azmacort	$60	Aventis
	Beclovent	$45	GlaxoSmithKline
	Flovent	$62	GlaxoSmithKline
	Pulmicort	$125	AstraZeneca
	Vanceril	$43	Schering
Cromolyn sodium	Intal	$72	Aventis
Nedocromil sodium	Tilade	$44	Aventis
Anti-leukotrienes	Accolate	$65	AstraZeneca
	Singulair	$82	Merck
	Zyflo	$97	Abbott
Theophylline	Theo-24	$20	UCB Pharma
	Theo-Dur	$37	Key
	Uni-dur	$36	Key
	Uniphyl	$31	Purdue Frederick
Combination	Advair (steroid and beta agonist)	$100	GlaxoSmithKline

*See appendix B for the phone numbers of the manufacturers.

As you can see from the table, there are many drugs in the different classes and their prices do vary. They can range from as low as $31 to as high as $125 for a month's supply. While these prices might not be the ones you will pay at your pharmacy, the differences in prices among the drugs will probably be the same. For those with insurance that covers prescription drugs, you will be able to use your copay to obtain the medications. You still will save on your medication if you used the mail-order operation of your insurer. Call your insurance company and ask how to go about doing that. Also, make sure you get the maximum refills from your doctor when sending in your script. This will save you on copays, and will reduce the chances of forgetting to get your refill.

If You Do Not Have Insurance

If you do not have insurance that covers medications, start by looking at patient assistance programs from drug companies. These programs give away free medicines to those who qualify. If you have a prescription for any of these products, call the company and see if you qualify for free medicines. If the company is not listed in appendix B, it means that they do not at this time have a patient assistance program.

Generic Substitutions

Some of the asthma medications are available as generics. A generic drug has the same active ingredient as the brand-name drug but is considerably less expensive. The following table shows the available generic equivalents.

Brand Name	Generic Name
Alupent	Metaproterenol
Intal	Cromolyn sodium
Proventil	Albuterol
Theo-24	Theophylline
Theo-Dur	Theophylline
Uni-dur	Theophylline
Uniphyl	Theophylline
Ventolin	Albuterol

Discuss with your physician and pharmacist the option of using a generic drug if that class of drug is available as a generic. Sometimes individuals might respond to a generic drug differently than they respond to a brand-name drug. If that is the case with you, be sure to let your doctor know.

Other programs for saving on medications include using discount pharmacy programs, Internet pharmacies, and state programs for those who qualify. See chapters 4 and 5 for these and other programs.

Hospitalization

Asthma is the number one cause of hospitalization for those between ages one and 17. Most asthmatics who show up in the hospital do so under emergency situations as their capacity to breathe becomes more and more restricted. Fortunately, the rate of dying from asthma in the hospital setting is very low. The problem is that of reaching emergency personnel before the attack becomes dangerous. *If you suspect an asthma attack and don't know what to do, call 911.* The longer you wait before getting help, the greater the chance of dying from the attack.

In dealing with the expense of hospitalization, insurance will cover the cost as defined by the policy. This will probably be true even if you go to an out-of-network facility because chances are you did so because it was an emergency. Medicaid pays for about a third of all asthma-related hospitalizations. Parents with low incomes should inquire about their Medicaid eligibility. Also, find out if your child qualifies for CHIP (Child Health Insurance Program), a government program designed for children under 19 years old who do not qualify for Medicaid.

If You Do Not Have Insurance

For those without insurance, if you have an asthma attack or suspect an asthma attack, do not think twice about calling the emergency service. The federal law that helps individuals without insurance will ensure that you get help at any facility. You might have to work out a payment plan later but the most important thing to realize is that an asthma attack is an emergency that can kill you. So get to the nearest hospital as quickly as possible.

Indirect Costs

Indirect costs in asthma come from workdays lost, time off from school, and cost related to the premature deaths of asthmatics. Lost productivity comes from individuals who are unable to work because they have to manage their asthma, as well as from parents and caregivers who have to miss work to care for the children who miss school or other functions because of their asthma. Some individuals also retire early because their asthma becomes a disability, affecting job performance.

Individuals with asthma have the full protection of the Americans with Disability Act (ADA). This means that an employer has to make reasonable accommodations so that the asthmatic can perform the essential functions of his or her job. The asthmatic should enjoy the full benefits that all other workers enjoy. In chapter 8, we described in detail these rights.

An important right that the ADA gives asthmatics is that of dealing with occupational asthma. If your working environment is exposing you to triggers that cause you to develop asthma attacks, you can request reasonable accommodations from the employer either to fix the problem or to move you to an environment free of the trigger. If your employer punishes you in any way because of this request, you have a legitimate case. Consult with an employment attorney.

Children with asthma and allergies are also protected by the ADA. This means that schools and other areas where children congregate must be supportive of the child with asthma, in both prevention as well as being able to administer the child's medication if an attack develops. Substances that are known allergens, such as dust, smoke, mold, and even nuts (like peanuts), should be avoided in an environment where a child is known to be allergic to them.

There is a huge industry designed to sell asthma-prevention products. While some of these can be truly helpful, most of them are a waste of money. A lot can be done to prevent asthma just by following the instructions listed in the prevention section. Most of these do not require spending money. If you think you need to take more precautions or are wondering about the usefulness of a particular product, call the Asthma and Allergy Foundation of America listed at the end of this chapter and they will advise you.

Complementary and Alternative Therapy

It must be stressed that when it comes to asthma, nonconventional medicine should be complementary and not alternative. This means that it is not advisable for a patient to forgo conventional treatment and use only nonconventional treatment. This is not because nonconventional treatments might not work, but rather because they have not been systematically studied. You cannot take chances with asthma because an acute attack can kill very quickly.

Complementary therapies used in conjunction with conventional therapies are usually designed to help with breathing and relaxation. Some of these include yoga, guided imagery, and deep breathing. Some spinal manipulations may also improve lung capacity. Certain herbs are thought to relax the airways but these have not been well studied and should never be used in an acute attack as alternatives to conventional medicines.

Resources

Allergy and Asthma
   Network/Mothers of
   Asthmatics
(800) 878-4403
www.aanma.org

American Academy of Allergy,
   Asthma, and Immunology
(800) 822-2762
www.aaaaai.org

American College of Allergy,
   Asthma and Immunology
(800) 842-7777
www.acaai.org

American Lung Association
(800) 586-4872
www.lungusa.org

Asthma and Allergy Foundation
   of America
(800) 727-8462
www.aafa.org

National Asthma Education and
   Prevention Programs
(310) 251-1222
www.nhlbi.nih.gov

CHAPTER 12

Cancer

C ancer is a disease that can affect nearly any part of the body. Each type of cancer is unique and the course of treatment varies, depending on the site and how far the cancer has progressed. This chapter provides an overview of cancer and the costs involved in managing it.

According to the National Cancer Institute, in 1997 there were about 9 million Americans alive with a history of cancer. Some of these individuals were considered cured while others still had evidence of existing cancer. In 2000, it was estimated that about 1.3 million new cases of cancer were diagnosed and that over half a million individuals died from cancer in that year alone. Cancer is therefore the second leading cause of death in the United States behind heart disease. One out of every four deaths in the United States is from cancer. For women between the ages of 35 and 75, cancer is the leading cause of death.

Progress in the fight against cancer is measured by the five-year relative survival rate, that is, people living five years after being diagnosed with cancer. At the present time, that number is 60 percent of all cancers combined. This means that just over half of the individuals diagnosed with cancer are still alive five years after being diagnosed.

What Is Cancer?

The body is made up of tiny structures called cells. Each tissue or organ has unique cells that give that structure its distinct characteristics. Thus we are made up of billions of many types of cells. These cells divide and grow as the body needs them. This is a normal process taking place in our bodies all the time and helps keep us healthy by making us grow and replacing old cells. We make what we need and get rid of what we don't need.

With cancer, however, this well-orchestrated cell growth gets out of control. Instead of a tissue or organ making just the number of cells it needs, the cells start multiplying out of control and these extra cells get big enough to form a mass called a tumor. There are two types of tumors: benign and malignant.

A benign tumor is one in which the mass of tissue is clearly defined and confined to an area. It is not considered a cancer. The cells in a benign tumor do not spread to other parts of the body. They can be more easily removed and usually do not grow back once removed. Benign tumors often are not considered life-threatening. They sometimes can be left alone if they stop growing and if the removal process is considered risky.

A malignant tumor, on the other hand, is a cancer and is made up of cells that divide uncontrollably and do not stick with each other as much as the normal cells in that area do. As these cells divide and grow, they are likely to break off from one another and invade neighboring areas or get into the blood stream or the lymphatic system, which is another transport system in the body. The cells are then carried to other areas, where they can lodge and continue growing, forming new masses. This spread from the original site to other areas is known as metastasis. Malignant tumors kill either by destroying the tissue or organ of origin or by spreading and destroying other organs.

Causes

Many factors are associated with causing cancer. Cancer, however, is a complex process and occurs over time. It is usually caused by a combination of inheritance, lifestyle, and environment. It is still not well understood why some people are more prone to getting cancer while others are not. Many individuals get cancer yet have no known risk factor.

The risk factors that have been identified with cancer are:

• Heredity, that is, family history of cancer
• Use of tobacco

- Exposure to ultraviolet (UV) radiation from the sun or other sources
- Certain viruses like the papillomavirus (cervical cancer) and cytomegalovirus (Kaposi's sarcoma)
- Ionizing radiation, from X rays and radioactive substances
- Certain chemicals and substances like asbestos, benzene, formaldehyde, nickel, pesticides, and uranium

Symptoms

Most cancers are usually without symptoms at the beginning of the growth and sometimes by the time you notice any symptoms, the cancer may have progressed to a very dangerous stage. However, certain signs and symptoms indicate that you should be examined by your doctor to rule out the possibility of cancer. These symptoms include:

- A lump or mass anywhere, especially the breast or testes
- Coughing that persists
- A sore that does not heal
- Changes in weight that cannot be determined
- Unusual bleeding
- Changes in bowel movement
- Changes in urinating
- Difficulty swallowing
- Changes in a wart or mole

Remember that many of these symptoms can be brought about by other diseases. So before deciding it is cancer, see your doctor for a more precise diagnosis.

Types

Nearly every part of the body is capable of producing cancer cells, so cancers are usually classified based on the part of the body from which they originate. The most common cancers are breast cancer, colon cancer, lung cancer, and prostate cancer.

Once cancer is detected, the doctor performs a "staging," which is the determination of the extent of the disease: how big the cancer is, whether it has spread, and if so to what other parts of the body. The results of the staging allow the doctor to determine if other tests are needed and what types of treatments should be used. The stages range from I (early stage) to IV (advanced stage).

Prevention

While you cannot change your genetic inheritance, other things can be done to prevent cancer. Environmental factors are believed to account for over half of all cancers. Let's examine some of the things that we can do to cut down on our chances of getting cancer.

Stopping Tobacco Use

Stopping the use of tobacco is the single most effective way to prevent death due to cancers. It is estimated that smoking accounts for at least one-third of all cancer deaths per year in the United States. The risk of getting lung cancer from smoking increases with the number of years one has been smoking, the type of tobacco product (some have more nicotine than others), and how deeply one inhales. Smoking also increases the chances of getting other cancers, like cancers of the mouth, throat, pancreas, bladder, kidney, and cervix.

The smoking of cigars and pipes also carries the risk of cancers of the mouth and throat. Secondhand smoke—that is, breathing the smoke from a smoker—can also increase your chance of getting lung cancer even if you are a nonsmoker.

The good news is that when you stop smoking, the risk of cancer begins to decrease, and this risk declines with every year you stay tobacco-free.

There are prescription medications and over-the-counter remedies to help individuals stop smoking. Many organizations and government agencies can also help. Many communities have support groups that help individuals stop smoking. To find out about the group in your area, call the Cancer Information Service (CIS), toll-free, at (800) 4-CANCER. CIS can also provide other resources to those struggling to kick the habit.

Avoiding Excess Alcohol Consumption

Heavy use of alcohol has also been associated with cancers of the mouth, throat, and liver, among others.

Eating a Healthy Diet

There is an association between high-fat diets and certain cancers such as colon, uterus, and prostate cancers. Being overweight has been linked to breast cancer among older women and to cancers of the prostate, uterus, colon, pancreas, and ovaries.

Conversely, foods high in fiber, fruits, and vegetables have been associated with low risks of cancer. They have been shown to decrease the risk of throat, mouth, stomach, colon, lung, and prostate cancers.

If you follow the guidelines on proper nutrition suggested in chapter 2, you will be on your way to achieving the type of nutritional state that may decrease your chances of getting many types of cancers.

Avoiding Cancer-Causing Environmental Factors

Since we know that many environmental factors increase our chances of getting cancer, we should minimize our exposure to these factors. Sunlight and artificial tanning lamps are two of those factors because of the UV rays that they produce. There are many things you can do to reduce your exposure to these rays:

- Reduce exposure to the midday sun (when there is a greater concentration of UV rays).
- Wear broad-brimmed hats.
- Wear protective clothing.
- Wear sunscreens. The higher the sun protection factor (SPF), the better. Between 12 and 29 is thought to be adequate.

A controversy is brewing in the medical community about whether hormone replacement therapy (HRT), especially when estrogen is used alone, increases the risk of cancer of the uterus and of the breast. To counter this effect some doctors use a combination of estrogen and another hormone called progesterone.

Managing the Cost of Cancer Treatment

According to the National Institutes of Health, the overall cost of managing cancer in 2000 was estimated at $180 billion. Of this, $60 billion was for direct medical costs, $15 billion for lost productivity due to illnesses, and $105 billion for loss of productivity due to premature death.

The most important aspect in controlling the cost of cancer is *early detection.* Early detection not only reduces the number of procedures that will be needed, but also increases your chances of getting cured.

Screening and Testing

During routine or specially scheduled physical exams, your physician will check for any lumps or growths and also examine your blood. Other tests include lab tests, X rays, and tests for any abnormalities. Certain parts of the body are specifically checked for cancer, usually based on your age:

Breasts. The National Cancer Institute suggests that women in their 40s and above get a yearly mammogram (an X ray that provides an image of the internal breast structures).

Cervix. The Pap smear is used to detect changes in the cervix that might lead to cancer. This is usually part of every examination by gynecologists.

Colon and rectum. People over the age of 50 need to be examined for the presence of colorectal cancer, especially if there is a family history of the disease.

Other parts of the body that might be routinely examined are: the prostate in men over 50; the lungs in those who smoke; the skin for those with long exposures to the sun or who are fair-skinned; and the ovaries in women.

When cancer is detected or suspected, the doctor usually asks for a series of other tests to confirm the initial diagnosis. These include imaging with X rays, CAT scans, ultrasound, and MRI. A biopsy (where a portion of the tissue is taken and examined under a microscope) will also be done. Additional lab tests are done to check for markers, the substances that distinguish each particular cancer.

If cancer is confirmed, a course of treatment is decided upon. The three main ways of treating cancer are surgery (to cut out the cancer), chemotherapy (drugs used to kill the cancer), and radiation (high-energy rays used to kill the cancer cells).

Other therapies—such as hormone therapy, immunotherapy, and bone-marrow transplants—can also be used. Before starting a course of treatment, it is advisable to get a second opinion. Some insurance companies actually require second opinions before they will cover the treatment, so check with your carrier.

Most of the diagnosis and treatment (including medications) of cancer takes place in the hospital. Thus, in dealing with the cost of taking care of cancer, closely review chapter 7. Following is some additional information that is specific to cancer.

If You Have Insurance

If you have insurance coverage, be sure to understand the coverage policy on cancer. This is important because a lot of cancers do not respond to standard therapy and physicians are always looking for new ways to fight cancer. A lot of times what your physician might do will be considered experimental by the insurance company, which might therefore refuse to pay for it. If you find yourself in this situation, your physician is your best advocate. He or she should make a strong case for why that was the best treatment available. In this regard, it is important to solicit the input of other physicians, especially those who are highly regarded in the treatment of that particular cancer. If this fails, you might want to call your state department of insurance (see appendix A) or your local government representative to intervene on your behalf.

Medicare patients should be relieved to know that while Medicare does not cover prescription drugs outside the hospital, it will cover any drug that your physician administers in his or her office. Most chemotherapies are administered in the physician's office and this is covered by Medicare.

If You Do Not Have Insurance

If you do not have insurance coverage and you are diagnosed with cancer, you should go to a hospital to get treated and worry about payment later. You can always arrange a payment plan with the hospital. Read chapter 7 to understand some of the options available to you.

Another resource at your disposal is to enroll in a clinical study. There are many government-funded and drug-company funded studies around the country and you are bound to find one. The study will pay for everything, sometimes including transportation. To find out where these studies are being conducted call the National Cancer Institute at (800) 4-CANCER, or log on to the web site at http://cancer.gov. This site provides general information about clinical trials and also gives detailed information about ongoing studies.

A word about medications: there are other medical issues that can arise in cancer patients. For example, many suffer from pain and depression as a result of their diagnosis and treatment. If medications for these conditions are necessary, see chapters 4 and 5 on how to save money on prescription drugs as well as chapter 13, "Depression and Anxiety," for specifics about some of the medications. And since many of the medications to manage cancer pain are controlled substances, discuss with your doctors what your options are.

Resources

Many organizations help and advocate for victims of cancer and there are support groups for those who have the disease and are in remission. You can find these in your local phone book. If you need more information or are in need of resources, there are two main places to go:

American Cancer Society
(800) ACS-2345
www.cancer.org

National Cancer Institute
(800) 4-CANCER
www.nci.nih.gov

CHAPTER 13

Depression and Anxiety

Mental disorders are common in the United States and around the world. The National Institute of Mental Health estimates that over 44 million North Americans suffer from mental illness in any one year. Two of the most common mental illnesses are depression and anxiety disorders. Depression affects over 18 million while over 19 million have an anxiety disorder. Mental illness is the second leading cause of disability and premature death, after heart disease.

What Is Depression?

Depression is a brain disorder. It can affect your thoughts, moods, feelings, behavior, and physical health. Unfortunately, many people still think it is "all in your head" and that if the person would only try harder, he or she could snap out of the depression. This is not true. Doctors now know that it is a medical disorder with a biological basis, just like diabetes or arthritis.

When we talk about depression, it is important to keep in mind that most people will experience some of the symptoms of depression during their lifetimes. It is natural to feel depressed when you lose a loved one, your marriage breaks up, or you are fired from your job. What distinguishes chronic depression from feeling sad about a situation is that depression affects your mood, bodily functions, and daily behavior, and it usually does not go away without treatment.

While a stressful life event can be the "trigger" for depression, many times depression occurs spontaneously without any identifiable, specific cause. Depression may occur as repeated episodes over a lifetime, with depression-free periods in between. Or it may be a chronic condition, requiring ongoing treatment over a lifetime. Typically, the first episode occurs between the ages of 25 and 44. It is more common in older people, but it is also more likely to go unrecognized in this age group. Depression rates are lower among married people (especially married men) and those in long-term relationships. It is higher among divorced people and those who live alone.

Recognizing depression is not always easy since depressed people often tend to withdraw from family and friends and isolate themselves. And when they go to a doctor, they don't complain that they are depressed. Instead, they talk about not being able to sleep, or having no energy. However, certain things that people may notice about themselves, or that someone else may notice about them, may be a sign that something is wrong.

Symptoms

Depression can contribute to a wide variety of other health problems, such as generalized itching, blurred vision, excessive sweating, dry mouth, gastrointestinal problems (indigestion, constipation, and diarrhea), headache, and backache. For a doctor to diagnose depression, you must have the following signs and symptoms most of the day, nearly every day, for at least two weeks.

The two main symptoms of depression are:

- Loss of interest in normal daily activities. You feel no interest or pleasure in activities that you used to enjoy, like sports.
- Depressed mood. You feel sad, helpless, and hopeless and may have crying spells.

If you have either one of these, as well as four or more of the following symptoms, you may be depressed:

- Significant weight loss or gain
- Sleep disturbances
- Fatigue
- Excessive restlessness
- Low self-esteem—feelings of worthlessness and excessive guilt
- Thoughts of death
- Impaired thinking or concentration

Complications

Depression is not easy to manage. Since many people still view mental illness as a character flaw or a personal weakness, people are often afraid to admit they have it and delay seeking treatment or do not get treated at all. If left untreated, short-term complications of depression can lead to long-term complications.

Short-term complications include:

- Feelings of sadness, fatigue, hopelessness
- Inability to enjoy family and friends
- Job troubles

Long-term complications include:

- Cardiovascular complications
- Substance abuse
- Hospitalization
- Loss of income
- Divorce
- Suicide

Depressed people don't usually follow healthy habits, including sensible diet and exercise. Studies have shown that people with depression suffer greater risk of heart disease than people who are not depressed.

The most dreaded complication of depression is suicide. Approximately 10 to 15 percent of patients hospitalized with depression commit suicide.

What Is Anxiety?

With anxiety, the person has an unpleasant emotional state accompanied by changes similar to those caused by fear. The state might arise suddenly or develop gradually over time. When these changes start affecting the person's ability to function and do not go away within a few days, the person may be suffering from an anxiety disorder. There are many types of anxiety disorders. The main types are:

- Panic disorder
- Obsessive-compulsive disorder

- Post-traumatic stress disorder
- Generalized anxiety disorder
- Phobias

Panic Disorder

People with panic attacks suffer from sudden attacks of fear. They often have a rapid heartbeat, sweating, feeling of choking, and fear of losing control, going crazy, or even dying. The attacks build up quickly and last for about 10 minutes. If these attacks persist and the individual is always concerned about having these attacks, they are considered to have a panic disorder.

Obsessive-Compulsive Disorder (OCD)

Some people with OCD have thoughts they can't get out of their head, such as that something bad is going to happen to them or a family member. Others feel compelled to act in order to prevent a dreaded event they think could happen if they don't perform a particular behavior. For example, people with OCD may wash their hands repeatedly to get rid of germs, or enact certain rituals such as counting or putting their books in alphabetical order.

We all have compulsions to some extent. Most of us have had the experience of wondering if we locked the door to our house or turned off the stove. But the person with OCD feels compelled to go back and check repeatedly. If such behavior starts being distressful and affects the quality of life, then the person might have OCD.

Post-traumatic Stress Disorder (PTSD)

Many years ago, it was first reported that soldiers had recurring nightmares about things they had seen during the war. In our society, people who have witnessed a traumatic event, whether it is the murder of a loved one or a violent crime, or have been involved in a traumatic event such as a plane crash, are often deeply affected by the experience. Many are haunted by images they cannot get out of their mind, suffer recurring dreams, or even feel that the event is happening to them again. People with this disorder often report trouble sleeping and difficulty concentrating, and are irritable and prone to attacks of anger.

Generalized Anxiety Disorder (GAD)

People with GAD suffer from excessive worry and anxiety for at least a six-month period. They are often restless, can't sleep, have difficulty concentrating, and experience muscle tension.

Phobias

Phobias can involve specific or general worries. Spiders may terrify one person, while another person fears being in public, open spaces. The person avoids any place or situation where there might be crowds or when help is unavailable in the event of developing sudden, panic-like symptoms. This is known as agoraphobia. People with agoraphobia refuse to leave their homes because they are afraid that they will have a panic attack if they do. Someone else may not be afraid of flying, but won't fly because he or she fears getting a panic attack on the plane.

People with social phobias avoid situations where they will be exposed to new situations or scrutiny by others. Giving a speech is a common fear of many people. Who wants to make a mistake or appear foolish to others? But when a person avoids *all* social situations out of fear of rejection and the feelings that it might bring, this can lead to a very lonely life.

Complications

Obviously, if you are feeling anxious, you are not feeling your best. Constantly being under stress, not sleeping well, and being afraid does not make for an ideal lifestyle. Those with OCD report that constantly checking and worrying about things leaves them exhausted. There is also a high correlation between anxiety and depression. Constant stress also can lead to cardiovascular complications. People with panic disorder and agoraphobia are at risk for suicide.

Short-term complications include:

- Uncomfortable feelings and symptoms
- Inability to enjoy life
- Anticipatory anxiety that leads to the cancelation of many activities

Long-term complications include:

- Cardiovascular complications
- Agoraphobia
- Inability to enjoy life
- Depression
- Increased risk of suicide

High-Risk Factors

Certain factors can increase the risk of someone developing depression or an anxiety disorder:

- *Heredity.* If you have parents or siblings with these conditions, you have a higher chance of developing an anxiety disorder than someone whose family does not have the conditions.
- *Female sex.* Women appear to develop depression more than men. It is not known if this is truly biological or if it is because women report these symptoms and seek help in far greater numbers than men do.
- *Stressors.* Significant events that create stress in one's life can lead to depression or an anxiety disorder. The death of a loved one can precipitate depression. Being in a war or surviving a plane crash can lead to an anxiety disorder.

Prevention

If any of these illnesses run in your family, there is a higher chance that a family member may develop it. So if you know your family history and you see a family member in trouble, you might be able to head off problems if he or she is diagnosed and treated right away.

There are no blood tests to detect depression or anxiety and no vaccinations against mental illness. The good news is that both depression and anxiety can be treated with medication, psychotherapy, or a combination of both.

Managing the Cost

The cost of mental illnesses to society is estimated to be $79 billion a year, with depression alone costing $44 billion.

Treatment for depression or anxiety comes in three forms: psychotherapy, medication, or a combination of both.

Psychotherapy

Both depression and anxiety can be treated without medication. Cognitive therapy, which helps a person to understand his or her patterns of thinking and behavior and how to change them, has proven just as effective as medication in both depression and panic disorder.

Medication

Medications offer quick relief and are faster than psychotherapy alone. It usually takes about two to six weeks for an antidepressant to be effective, while psychotherapy can take years to achieve an effect. Some patients do need medication to put their mental health back in balance.

Combination of Psychotherapy and Medication

Since psychiatric illnesses may have both biological and psychological components, there are issues that you might want to talk to a therapist about, even if you get better from medication alone.

Direct Costs

The direct costs of managing these mental disorders come from visits to a health professional, medications, and hospitalization.

Visits to a Health Professional

If you or a loved one has symptoms of anxiety or depression, it is important to get a diagnosis and know what you are dealing with. A good place to start is with your family physician, because another illness, such as a thyroid disorder, could be the underlying cause rather than a mental illness. Once any underlying physical disorder is ruled out, a treatment plan can be made.

Many family physicians are now trained to diagnose both depression and anxiety in their patients and can start you on a medication or refer you to a therapist. If you have insurance, you will only have to pay the copay for the visit, which ranges from $5 to $20 depending on your plan. However, if your doctor feels that you need to see a mental health professional, you should try to see someone who is in your plan. If you do not, you will have to pay a lot of money since most plans do not cover out-of-network mental health professional visits.

The diagnosis and treatment of mental illness is an art and not necessarily an exact science. It combines both medical issues and psychological issues. Most research has shown that a combination of medication and psychotherapy has the best results over the long term.

Your primary care physician might not have the time or the training to administer psychotherapy. Psychotherapy can be received from psychiatrists, who are M.D.s; clinical psychologists, who are Ph.D.s; or social workers, who usually have a master's degree and are certified by the state. Many people believe that it is best to get your medication and therapy from the same person, but only an M.D. can prescribe drugs. Some states are looking at giving psychologists the power to prescribe. New Mexico became the first state to do this and other states are likely to follow.

Insurance companies do not treat mental illness the same as they do a physical illness. Most insurance companies pay only 50 percent of the cost of psychotherapy, or limit the number of visits. Many insurance companies also make it prohibitively expensive if you see a doctor outside their network of providers.

In most HMO plans, you need a referral to a mental health professional. Very often the system is administered by another separate organization (called a carve-out), which specializes in mental health. As long as you see their network of providers, you will only have to pay a copay. However, sometimes you have little choice of whom you see and the number of visits is restricted, often to about 30 a year.

If you are not in an HMO your insurance company will cover the cost of seeing a mental health professional. But they usually do not reimburse you for the 80 percent as they do for doctor's visits. They also limit the number of visits a year.

Remember, who you see for therapy is very important. You need to see someone whom you can talk to and whom you trust. If the only person you can find this bond with is not in the network, it might be worth spending the extra money for treatment. Don't forget that Medicare includes mental health coverage.

When choosing a therapist, keep in mind:

- Is this person covered by my plan?
- If I choose to see someone not on the plan, how long can I afford to see this person?

Also, keep in touch with your family doctor, especially if you are on medication. When you are on certain medications, you may need to have certain tests done periodically.

If You Do Not Have Insurance

If you do not have insurance, remember that most communities have public and private clinics that offer treatment either for free or on a sliding scale based on your income. More than $12 billion from state and local government and more than $1 billion from federal government block grant and Veteran Affairs funds were given to cover mental health services for the uninsured. If you have to pay for treatment, realize that psychiatrists are the most expensive mental health professionals. Social workers are the least costly. If you find a good social worker for therapy, he or she can work with your primary care physician or a psychiatrist to obtain medication for you.

Medications

You should always start with one medication, known as monotherapy. This cuts down on chances of side effects, and also reduces your medication costs. If one drug fails to achieve desired relief then another drug can be added.

The following tables show the different classes of drugs that can be used to manage depression and anxiety and their manufacturers. The prices of these drugs vary considerably from a low of about $25 to a high of about $93 a month for medications for depression, and between $25 and $95 a month for anxiety medications. So talk to your doctor about starting with a less expensive one unless there is a reason not to.

The table below lists prescription drugs used to manage depression, as well as the manufacturers of those drugs.

Class	Brand Names	Cost of a Month's Starting Dose	Manufacturer*
Tricyclics	Elavil	$25	AstraZeneca
	Norpramin	$70	Aventis
	Pamelor	$110	Mallinckrodt
	Tofranil	$50	Mallinckrodt
Serotonin-Specific Reuptake Inhibitors (SSRI)	Celexa	$65	Forest
	Paxil	$72	GlaxoSmithKline
	Prozac	$80	Lilly
	Zoloft	$65	Pfizer
Monoamine oxidase inhibitors	Nardil	$50	Pfizer
	Parnate	$65	GlaxoSmithKline
Others	Desyrel	$93	Apothecon
	Effexor XR	$67	Wyeth
	Remeron	$77	Organon
	Serzone	$76	Bristol-Myers Squibb
	Wellbutrin SR	$47	GlaxoSmithKline

*See appendix B for the phone numbers of the manufacturers.

The following drugs are used to manage anxiety.

Class	Brand Names	Cost of a Month's Starting Dose	Manufacturer*
Benzodiazepines	Ativan	$32	Wyeth
	Klonopin	$25	Roche
	Serax	$80	Faulding
	Xanax	$68	Pharmacia
	Valium	$37	Roche
Serotonin-Specific Reuptake Inhibitors (SSRI)	Luvox	$95	Solvay
	Paxil	$82	GlaxoSmithKline
	Zoloft	$62	Pfizer
Other	Buspar	$65	Bristol-Myers Squibb
	Effexor XR	$67	Wyeth

*See appendix B for the phone numbers of the manufacturers.

Generic Substitution

The following drugs are available as generics. If you are prescribed the brand name, ask your pharmacist to call your doctor to request the generic brand. The difference in cost can be substantial.

Brand Name	Generic Name
Ativan	Lorazepam
Desyrel	Trazadone
Elavil	Amitriptyline
Klonopin	Clonazepam
Nardil	Phenelzine
Norpramin	Desipramine
Pamelor	Nortriptyline
Parnate	Tranylcypromine
Prozac	Fluoxetine
Serax	Oxazepam
Tofranil	Imipramine
Valium	Diazepam
Xanax	Alprazolam

Pill Cutting

A lot of the drugs for depression and anxiety are available in different strengths. The prices are usually the same for the different strengths, so if you are at a lower dose, ask your doctor to prescribe the higher dose and then split it. Initially, ask for assistance from your pharmacist to make sure you are splitting the pill correctly. The savings in the long run can be substantial: you can actually cut your cost in half.

Drug Company Assistance Programs

The preceding tables identified the various drugs for depression and anxiety and their manufacturers. If you have been prescribed any of these products and you cannot afford them, call the manufacturer's number and explain your situation. If you need help in navigating the process, call one of the companies listed in chapter 5 for assistance. If a manufacturer is not listed in appendix B, that manufacturer did not offer a patient assistance program at the time of this writing.

Other Strategies to Reduce the Cost of Medications

Go back to chapters 4 and 5 and revisit the following strategies: mail order, discount pharmacy programs, the Internet, and/or state government programs. Use as many as you can. The more programs you use, the more savings you will achieve.

Hospitalization

Depression is the number one reason for hospitalization for those age 18 to 44. For all ages, it is the eighth reason behind all hospitalizations. Depression leads to such high rates of hospitalization because it is the number one risk for suicide; thus a person who is severely depressed needs to be closely monitored and treated. The issues related to the cost of hospitalization for depression and anxiety are the same as those discussed in chapter 7. Review that chapter as it relates to managing the cost of hospitalization with or without insurance. It should be noted that even though insurance companies sometimes treat mental disorders different from other disorders, there are Mental Health Parity Laws designed to make insurance companies treat mental health disorders equally.

Employment Issues

If you have depression or an anxiety disorder, you may be worried about the effect it might have on your job. The Supreme Court has held that having a mental illness can qualify one as being disabled and hence protected under the Americans with Disabilities Act (ADA). This protection covers hiring, firing, promotion, pay, and other benefits. The ADA covers only private employers. The Rehabilitation Act of 1973 covers government employees, and any employer who receives federal money is prohibited from discriminating against people with disabilities.

The Family and Medical Leave Act of 1993 allows you to take up to 12 weeks of unpaid leave each year to care for yourself or a family member with a serious illness. If the complication of your mental disorder requires time off to deal with it, this law ensures that you do not lose your job.

To help ensure that your disease is not affecting your work performance, it requires that you plan ahead. Pay attention to special circumstances that could affect you. This includes traveling, working odd hours, or attending long meetings. Remember that if you are on medication, there may be side effects to cope with at work. Some drugs make your mouth dry, so be sure to have lozenges or water if you go to a meeting. If a drug makes you tired at a particular point in the day, try to arrange your schedule so you do not have important meetings or work that requires intense concentration during those times.

Intangible Costs

Since the duration of a psychiatric illness is unpredictable, it can cause great stress on the family, especially when family members don't understand the person's behavior. Having a mental illness can cost you your friends, your job, and even your marriage. When a person is hospitalized for mental illness, family members often don't know what to say to others. But the worst intangible is suicide, which has a devastating effect on a family.

Family members or loved ones are usually the first ones to notice changes in an individual, either when they start developing a mental illness or when they start recovering from one. The support of relatives is very crucial to the recognition and recovery of those with mental illness. It can be emotionally draining on loved ones but the more they know about the disease and how to help, the less the impact the disease will have on everybody and the faster the recovery. So talk to your friends and relatives if you are suffering from depression.

Complementary and Alternative Remedies

According to the National Institute of Health's National Center for Complementary and Alternative Medicine (NCCAM), the U.S. Agency for Health Care Policy and Research, and other researchers, the following alternative therapies have been used to help individuals manage the symptoms of depression and anxiety.

Acupuncture

Many patients who are depressed and/or anxious report chronic pain, especially back pain. Acupuncture is recognized as an effective help for stress, tiredness, and anxiety. Patients usually feel better within the first four treatments, but some complex problems may take longer to clear. Acupuncture works in stages and will build in successive sessions. The use of acupuncture can be less expensive than the management of the pain through conventional therapy, especially for those not covered by insurance. Many insurers, however, are beginning to cover the costs of acupuncture if performed by a licensed acupuncturist.

Biofeedback

Biofeedback has been used to help individuals become more aware of their body's response to the signals caused by anxiety. This allows the individual to better manage and deal with such signals as pain and to better deal with stress. It is a powerful relaxation technique.

Other Behavioral Approaches

Depression and/or anxiety can cause insomnia, or not sleeping well. Relaxation and behavioral techniques corresponding to those used for chronic pain may also be used for specific types of insomnia. The following approaches can help manage insomnia:

- Restrict all activities in the bedroom except sleep and sex.
- Try not to fall asleep. Very often trying not to sleep causes the person to fall asleep.

Dr. Andrew Weil, a best selling author and director of the Program in Integrative Medicine at the University of Arizona in Tucson, says the best way to treat anxiety disorders is through breathing exercises. He also feels that 30 minutes of vigorous aerobic exercise will help treat depressed patients. For both depression and anxiety he also believes that following a healthy diet and using certain supplements can help.

Alternative Medicines

Many patients who take antidepressants report unpleasant side effects such as a dry mouth, nausea, headache, diarrhea, or impaired sexual function or sleep. Because of these side effects, many patients with depression are turning to herbal treatments. The most well known and studied is St. John's wort. Researchers are studying it for the possibility that it may have fewer and less severe side effects than conventional antidepressant drugs. St. John's wort costs far less than antidepressant medication and does not require a prescription. Clinical trials have found a similar rate of response with St. John's wort as with standard, conventional antidepressants in treating mild to moderate depression. When depression is severe, however, alternative therapies might not be as effective.

As with any complementary or alternative medicine use, let your physician know what you are taking since these herbs can interact with prescription drugs. Also if you are not getting better on these herbs alone, you should seek conventional help because if your mental disease is not adequately treated, the results can be catastrophic, leading to death.

Resources

American Psychiatric Association
(202) 682-6220
www.psych.org

American Psychological
  Association
(202) 336-5500
www.apa.org

Anxiety Disorders Association
  of America
(301) 231-9350
www.adaa.org

National Alliance for the
  Mentally Ill
(800) 950-NAMI (950-6264)
www.nami.org

National Center for PTSD
U.S. Department of Veterans
  Affairs
116D VA Medical and Regional
  Office Center
(802) 296-5132
www.ncptsd.org

National Depressive and
  Manic-Depressive
  Association
(800) 826-3632
www.ndmda.org

National Institute of Mental
  Health
(301) 443-4513
www.nimh.nih.gov

National Mental Health
  Association
(800) 969-NMHA (969-6642)
www.nmha.org

Obsessive Compulsive (OC)
  Foundation
(203) 315-2190
www.ocfoundation.org

CHAPTER 14

Diabetes

D iabetes is one of the most expensive and prevalent diseases known. It affects over 16 million individuals in the United States and about one-third of those affected are not even aware that they have the disease. Each year about 800,000 more people are diagnosed with diabetes. One estimate shows that the prevalence of diabetes in the population is expected to almost double by the year 2025. The aging of the population and an increase in obesity are the leading causes of this increase.

Diabetes is the fourth leading cause of death by disease in the United States, and its effects on the individual who has the disease, as well as those associated with the patient, are vast. Because most individuals with diabetes can live with the disease for a very long time after it is diagnosed, it can have a tremendous effect on both the individual's physical health and financial well-being. The good news is that careful management of the disease can reduce the stress of these complications and result not only in living a healthy and normal life, but also in preventing the cost from taking a big toll on individuals, their loved ones, and society as a whole.

What Is Diabetes?

Diabetes occurs when the body cannot control the amount of sugar in the blood. When we eat, the body turns most of the food into glucose, which is a form of sugar. This sugar provides the energy for the body to work. Normally, the amount of glucose in the blood is transported with the help of a chemical called insulin, which is produced by an organ near the stomach called the pancreas. Insulin is like a gatekeeper. It opens up our muscles and other tissues so that the glucose can get in to be used as needed. Excess glucose is stored in the liver and muscle until the need arises.

The body tries to keep the amount of glucose in the blood at a steady level. So if the amount of glucose goes up, as it does after a meal, the pancreas will secrete insulin, which then helps transport the glucose into the liver and muscle for storage and use. This brings the level of glucose back down to normal. If the amount of glucose is falling either because it is being used up or because of lack of eating, the body increases the amount of glucose in the blood in part by decreasing the amount of insulin that is secreted.

Diabetes occurs when the pancreas cannot make enough insulin or the pancreas makes insulin but the body cannot use the insulin effectively. When this happens, the glucose that the individual produces after eating does not get transported into muscles and other tissues effectively and hence the amount of glucose in the blood rises. The body now has a large amount of glucose circulating in the blood. Some of the glucose is actually sent out in the urine, which should not happen in normal circumstances.

Symptoms

Diabetes is one of the "silent killers." An individual can go for years with increased blood glucose and have no idea that he or she is diabetic because there might be no symptoms or the symptoms are mild and are not accompanied by pain and thus are ignored.

Unfortunately, when our glucose levels go up, the body does nothing to alert us immediately that our blood glucose is high. Everybody has changes in blood glucose levels because events such as eating and exercising affect these levels. Our bodies are constantly working to bring glucose levels back to normal. Only when the body can no longer maintain a normal glucose level is the individual diagnosed with diabetes. Over a long period of time, usually years, this increased blood glucose destroys different parts of the body and results in various complications.

The body gives signals to indicate that it might be suffering from diabetes. If you notice some or all of these symptoms, consult a health-care professional, who can determine if you have diabetes.

Symptoms that may arise from having diabetes are:

- Excessive thirst
- Constant urination, including unusual bedwetting in children
- Excessive hunger
- Weight loss despite eating
- Frequent tiredness
- Unusual vomiting
- Blurred vision
- Wounds that do not heal
- Loss of feeling or tingling in the hands and feet
- Dry and itchy skin

Having any one or a combination of these symptoms does not mean you have diabetes. But feeling these symptoms over a period of time should prompt you to seek medical advice.

Types

There are three types of diabetes: type 1 diabetes, type 2 diabetes, and gestational diabetes.

Type 1 Diabetes

Type 1 diabetes occurs when the pancreas does not produce enough insulin. It is therefore often referred to as insulin-dependent diabetes. About 10 to 15 percent of all people with diabetes have type 1, which is the most common type in people under 30 years old but may occur at any age. The symptoms of type 1 diabetes occur over a short period of time and if not diagnosed and treated with insulin can result in a life-threatening diabetic coma.

Type 2 Diabetes

In type 2 diabetes, the individual produces insulin but for reasons that are still not clearly known, the body no longer uses the insulin effectively. This is known as insulin resistance. The body tries to make even more insulin to compensate for the reduced effectiveness and eventually starts running out of insulin-producing capacity and the individual becomes like a type 1 diabetic, needing insulin.

While type 2 diabetes usually occurs in adults 40 years and older and is most common in adults 55 years and older, more and more teenagers are being diagnosed with it. About 85 to 90 percent of all people with diabetes have type 2. Most people with type 2 are overweight.

The symptoms of type 2 diabetes develop gradually, unlike those of type 1. It is therefore difficult, especially in the early stages, to know if someone has type 2 diabetes simply by looking for symptoms. The only way to find out is to be tested. Hence it is recommended that individuals in categories with a high risk for developing diabetes get routine tests to ensure that they are not diabetic. These high-risk groups are:

- Those who are obese.
- Those with close family members who have diabetes.
- Members of high-risk ethnic groups: African Americans, Hispanics, Native Americans, and Asians.
- Those with high blood pressure.
- Those with high cholesterol.
- Those with high glucose levels on a previous testing.

Gestational Diabetes

About 2 to 5 percent of pregnant women develop diabetes, which usually disappears after the child is born. Certain groups are considered more likely to develop gestational diabetes, including African Americans, Hispanics, Native Americans, and those with a family history of diabetes.

Although gestational diabetes resolves after giving birth, individuals who develop it should be monitored closely because they are at an increased risk for developing type 2 diabetes at a later stage in their lives.

Prevention

There are two types of prevention in diabetes, primary prevention and secondary prevention. In primary prevention, the goal is to prevent getting diabetes at all. While this might not be possible with type 1 diabetes, it is potentially possible to prevent type 2. In secondary prevention, the goal is to prevent the complications from developing when an individual has already been diagnosed with diabetes.

Primary Prevention

There are two main ways to prevent diabetes: diet and exercise.

As discussed in chapter 2, a healthy lifestyle can prevent a lot of illnesses, and that is very true when it comes to diabetes. Healthy living should be incorporated in the lifestyle of every individual, but if you are in the categories of individuals with a high risk for developing diabetes as mentioned previously, a healthy lifestyle is essential to prevent developing diabetes.

The single most important aspect in preventing the onset of diabetes is weight control. The more overweight an individual is, the greater the chances of developing diabetes. In one study, women who gained an excess 15 pounds over their usual weight increased their chances of developing diabetes by 50 percent.

Simple things you can do to lose weight include:

- Reduce the amount of food you eat, especially high-calorie foods like fats and simple sugars.
- Substitute fresh food for processed foods, which tend to have large amounts of salt, sugar, and fats.
- Reduce your stress level, which can lead to poor nutrition or overeating.
- Reduce your alcohol intake, since alcohol has a lot of calories with little nutritional value.
- Increase your activity level by choosing exercise in any form that you find enjoyable and can sustain.

Secondary Prevention

At this stage, you now have the disease and the goal is to make sure the complications that will be discussed later do not arise. This requires very tight management of the disease by following your doctor's orders. You must do everything you can to keep your sugar controlled through diet, exercise, and medication. The only way you can know that your sugar is controlled is by monitoring it as recommended by your doctor.

Diabetes prevention, both primary and secondary, is thought to be such powerful tools in managing the disease that nearly every health insurance company has a diabetes disease management program designed to help individuals with the disease learn more about it and how to control it effectively. Among health insurance companies it is one of the most managed of all the diseases, largely because the complications that develop can be very expensive.

Managing the Cost

The yearly cost of managing diabetes in the United States was estimated in 1997 to be $98 billion. It is important to understand that the primary goal is to obtain the most effective control of the disease while eliminating unnecessary costs. It cannot be overemphasized that very tight management of blood glucose level can significantly reduce the complications of diabetes, resulting in significant cost savings. The more complicated the disease is allowed to get, the more difficult it will be to treat and the more expensive it will become to manage. The most cost-effective way to manage diabetes is to prevent it from happening in the first place or, when it has occurred, to prevent the complications.

The costs are categorized into three groups: direct, indirect, and intangible costs.

Direct Costs

Direct costs come from:

- Physician visits and tests to manage the diabetes
- Management of the complications, including hospitalizations
- Medications

Physician Visits and Tests

When you start experiencing the symptoms of diabetes, you must be tested. If it turns out to be diabetes, get it seriously under control, because that is the best way to decrease the complications and reduce the costs. The first step is to see a healthcare professional, usually a doctor. After you are diagnosed with diabetes, it is important to realize that this might be a life-long illness, requiring your physician to monitor you on an ongoing basis. Frequent physician visits can be costly, not only in having to pay the physician for every visit but also in lost time from your job or from other activities that you could have been doing and enjoying more. To reduce the number of physician visits, it is important to ask your doctor as many questions as you can during the initial visit to understand what you need to do to control the disease and what types of unusual things might occur when you start therapy. You also need to provide your doctor with as much information as you can about your lifestyle, because this may help the doctor tailor a program for you and let you know what exactly you need to modify.

Make sure these topics are part of your conversation with your doctor:

- Your medical history (whether you have or have had any other diseases)
- Your family history of diseases, especially diabetes
- Your current lifestyle (eating, drinking, smoking, drug use)
- Exercise history
- Whether you are taking any medications
- Frequency of required blood glucose checks
- Possible side effects of medications
- Ways of gauging that your glucose is under control

Never be shy about calling your doctor if you have questions about your disease state or your treatment. Many visits can be saved by clearly following your doctor's advice and calling with questions about things you might be experiencing.

Your doctor will give you two types of tests:

- Tests to diagnose for diabetes
- Tests to determine how well the treatment is controlling your diabetes

Tests for Diagnosis

Basically, one test is done to determine if you have diabetes. This is called the fasting plasma glucose (FPG) test. It requires that blood be taken from the patient after an overnight fast and checked for the level of glucose. Normal glucose levels are less than 115 mg/dl for an adult and less than 130 mg/dl for a child. Don't worry about the mg/dl—that is a unit of measurement. The important thing is to remember the numbers themselves. If the glucose level is over 126 for an adult and over 140 for a child on two occasions, that person should seek follow-up for diabetes care.

Your doctor might decide to do another test called the oral glucose tolerance test (OGTT). This test is helpful if the glucose level is between 115 and 140 and if the individual is exhibiting the symptoms of diabetes discussed previously. This test is not as reliable as the FPG test since other factors, such as medications and age, can affect the result.

The FPG test is less expensive and more reliable than the OGGT test. So unless your doctor has another reason for doing one, there is no need to do an OGGT. The FPG can be done at the doctor's office and thus there are no costs of using outside laboratories.

Tests to Monitor Control

Once you have been diagnosed with diabetes, the single most important aspect in managing the disease is to keep a tight control on your blood glucose level. Several large studies have shown that an individual who maintains good control over blood glucose can significantly avoid the complications of diabetes. The two tests done to determine blood sugar levels during treatment are the finger-stick test and the Hb A1C test.

The finger-stick test is usually done at home. This is known as self-monitoring of blood glucose (SMBG). The patient obtains a small amount of blood, usually by pricking the finger, and then measures the blood glucose using a monitor that has a strip or cartridge to absorb the blood. The guidelines for SMBG testing are:

Type 1. Test before each meal and at bedtime. Also test two hours after breakfast and dinner.

Type 2. Test twice a day as needed to reach the goal glucose level. Test at different times to get a better sense of your average glucose level. If you are on insulin, you might be instructed to test more than twice a day.

If you have health insurance, call your doctor and schedule a visit. The cost for this visit is usually your copay. If you have indemnity insurance, you will usually pay 20 percent and the plan 80 percent of the fees deemed allowable, which would include the doctor's visit.

Most HMO plans allow the copay only if you see your primary care physician. If you decide to see a physician outside the plan's network or visit a specialist without getting a referral from your primary care physician, your plan would most likely make you pay nearly all of the cost of that visit. Diabetes is a disease that can easily be diagnosed by a primary care physician and except in the case of a diabetic coma, does not rise to being an emergency. So, to be cost-wise, schedule an appointment with your primary care physician first instead of with a specialist. If you need to see a specialist, usually an endocrinologist (a doctor who specializes in metabolic diseases, of which diabetes is one), or a nephrologist (a specialist in kidney diseases), your primary care physician can make that determination.

Home testing is so critical that Medicare and Medicaid pay for the equipment that the patient needs. Most insurance companies also pay for this home testing. At the time of this writing, all states except Alabama, Idaho, Montana, North Dakota, Ohio, and Oregon have laws governing the payment for diabetes testing equipment. In essence, the laws state that any insurance company licensed in the state to provide health insurance must reimburse patients for diabetes equipment, supplies, and education that the doctor has deemed medically necessary to help manage their diabetes. If you have insurance, inquire about the payment policy on home testing.

If You Do Not Have Health Insurance

If you are experiencing the symptoms of diabetes, it is extremely important to get a diagnosis because early detection will save you money. If you do not have health insurance there are ways to still get tested. One is to call advocacy groups such as the American Diabetes Association (see below for organizations and phone numbers) and ask for centers in your area where you can get tested for free. Another way to get a free test is to go to a community center, a church, or a health fair program that is giving free testing. Health fairs almost always provide tests for diabetes.

Another way is to investigate whether there are any federally funded clinics in the area. These clinics provide services for reduced fees and accept payments on a sliding scale based on income. If these are not available, the last alternative is to call physicians and let them know that you think you might have diabetes and you need a diagnosis. Remember to call only primary care physicians (internists or family doctors) and not specialists, who are more expensive.

What if you do not have health coverage or your insurance does not cover the cost of home testing? If you have diabetes, home testing is a must. To reduce your cost you should realize that the most expensive aspect of home testing is buying the strips (you need a new one each time you test yourself) and not the machine itself, which is a one-time cost. In fact, a lot of manufacturers make the machine available at a deep discount through retailers. So shop around for the prices of strips. Local pharmacies are always having promotions on glucose testing products—take advantage of these. A service called the Diabetic Supply Grant program assists individuals with diabetic supplies; it is administered by Crystal Home Care. If you are having financial difficulties with your diabetic supplies, call them at (800) 493-4902.

Managing the Complications

What makes diabetes so costly to manage is the fact that it affects so many parts of the body. It is also (with the exception of gestational diabetes) a life-long condition, which means that it has to be managed for very long periods. Without proper management, it can result in both short-term and long-term complications.

Short-term complications include low blood sugar, also known as hypoglycemia, and diabetic coma, also known as ketoacidosis.

Hypoglycemia

When the level of blood glucose falls too low because of medications, exercise, or not eating, the individual will become hypoglycemic (experience low blood sugar), becoming nervous, shaky, and confused, and perhaps even fainting. Functioning becomes impaired. This is usually corrected by rapidly eating some sugar.

Ketoacidosis

When the glucose in the blood cannot get into the tissues because of insufficient insulin, the body starts breaking down fats to generate energy, resulting in waste products called ketones. The body tries to get rid of the ketones through the urine but since the ketones build up and the body cannot get rid of them as fast as they are formed, they accumulate in the blood. Some are eliminated through the lungs. For reasons still not known, these ketones can dull the brain and cause coma, which can be life-threatening. Coma arising from high blood glucose is therefore referred to as diabetic ketoacidosis.

Long-term complications include:

• Cardiovascular complications
• Eye disease

- Foot amputation
- Kidney disease
- Nerve damage

Cardiovascular Complications

People with diabetes develop cardiovascular diseases two to four times more often than people without diabetes. Their risk of developing stroke is about two and a half times as high as without diabetes. Cardiovascular diseases are the leading cause of disability and death in people with type 2 diabetes.

Eye Disease

Diabetes is the leading cause of blindness in individuals age 20 and older. About 2 percent of all individuals who have had diabetes for 15 years or more become blind and about 10 percent develop severe damage to their eyesight, resulting in blurred vision.

Foot Amputation

Each year about 55,000 amputations are performed in individuals with diabetes. Diabetes is the leading cause of the loss of limbs besides being in an accident. These amputations occur because the limbs have been severely damaged from poor blood circulation and nerve damage. It starts with loss of sensation in the limbs leading to poor weight-bearing postures. The individual is also likely to begin using ill-fitting shoes because the lack of sensation means the person can't tell that the shoes are too tight. Eventually, infections develop that do not heal properly. The limb becomes severely damaged and the only way to prevent further damage is to cut it off.

Kidney Disease

Diabetes is a leading cause of kidney failure. About 10 percent to 20 percent of people with diabetes develop kidney diseases, leading to dialysis or kidney transplant. The numbers are even worse for individuals with type 1 diabetes; it is estimated that about 40 percent of individuals with type 1 diabetes develop severe kidney disease by age 50.

Nerve Damage

Diabetes can damage the nerves in many parts of the body. In the limbs, this can result in tingling sensations, numbness, and severe deep-seated pain. When the nerves on the blood vessels are damaged, the individual will experience fainting, poor bladder function, poor stomach movements, and impotence. At least half of all diabetics experience some form of nerve damage, or what is clinically called diabetic neuropathy.

As diabetes progresses, complications start developing. The poorer the sugar control, the quicker the complications appear and the more severe they will become. There is no clear order in which they appear; they are different in different individuals. The three ways of dealing with complications are:

- Through medications
- In an outpatient setting
- Through inpatient hospitalization

The complications that can be managed largely through medications are:

- Cardiovascular complications, including such illnesses as high blood pressure and high cholesterol
- Sexual dysfunction
- Pain

Because your primary care physician can manage the treatments for these conditions, the cost is relatively low. See chapters 4 and 5 for how to save money on prescription drugs.

The following complications can be managed on an outpatient basis; that is, you see a specialist who performs a procedure, but you get to go home the same day.

- Eye diseases
- Dialysis to assist the damaged kidney

Because medical procedures are now involved, the cost starts getting higher. See chapter 6 for strategies on how to reduce these costs.

As the diabetes worsens, certain conditions develop that require hospital stays, including:

- Severe cases of hypo- or hyperglycemia
- Diabetic coma
- Amputations
- Kidney transplant

At this point, the costs are going through the roof.

The strategies for dealing with all these costs rest largely on what you have to deal with. If you have insurance coverage, you will likely be covered for nearly all of the complications, but you must pay attention to your copays and deductibles. Remember, the more visits you make to the doctor, the more out-of-pocket costs you will incur. And always check your policy before getting any procedures so that you can plan financially. Be especially careful if you have managed care: make sure that you do not use a specialist without the appropriate referral. As the complications move on to in-patient care and hospitalization, you will need more and more specialists. They are more expensive, so do not go out of your plan's network unless you absolutely must. Check to make sure that a physician or hospital is in your plan's network and that you have followed the plan's procedures before getting the services.

If You Do Not Have Insurance

If you do not have insurance and you develop diabetes, explore every means of acquiring health insurance before any complications develop. Diabetes is one of the most expensive diseases to manage because there are so many complications, some of which require expensive procedures. If you wait for a complication to develop, you will end up paying higher premiums—if you can find any plan to accept you. Review chapter 1 on ways to get health insurance and explore your eligibility for them.

If you start needing care, be even more careful about using specialists. Always start with a primary care physician and get as much done as you can with that doctor. Only when he or she has determined that you absolutely need to see a specialist should you do so. Check out the different options mentioned in chapter 7 for dealing with institutional costs. This includes using outpatient facilities like urgicenters and surgicenters before using hospitals. If you have to use a hospital, start with public hospitals if possible, since specialized centers are usually more expensive.

Explore government programs. Diabetes is one of those diseases that are considered so serious that the government has set up programs to help individuals deal with it. Medicare, for example, although designed for seniors (those 65 and older), also takes care of those with end-stage renal disease, one of the complications of diabetes. So check with your state's health department for assistance or call the American Diabetes Association (ADA) at (800) 342-2383 for assistance. Besides the ADA, other advocacy groups listed at the end of the chapter can help you with the various complications. Call them for help.

Medications

If diet and exercise fail to control your blood glucose, the next step is to add medications. You should always start with one medication, which is called monotherapy. This cuts down on the chances of side effects, but it also reduces your medication costs. If one drug fails to achieve goal glucose levels, then another drug can be added. Let's examine some of the techniques that can be used to achieve savings with drugs for diabetes.

Brand-Name Substitution

The following table shows the different classes of drugs that can be used to manage blood sugar levels. The prices vary considerably, from a low of about $10 to a high of about $95 or more for a month's supply. While prices may be different in your neighborhood, the range of prices and the spread between different drugs are likely going to stay the same. So talk to your doctor about starting with a less expensive drug unless there is a reason not to.

Class	Brand Names	Cost of a Month's Starting Dose	Manufacturer*
Insulins	Humalog	$45	Lilly
	Novolin	$26	Novo Nordisk
	Velosulin	$33	Novo Nordisk
Alpha-Glucosidase Inhibitors	Precose	$50	Bayer
	Glyset	$52	Pharmacia
Sulfonlyureas	Amaryl	$10	Aventis
	Diabenese	$22	Pfizer
	DiaBeta	$11	Aventis
	Glucotrol XL	$11	Pfizer
	Glynase PresTabs	$17	Pharmacia
	Micronase	$15	Pharmacia

(continued)

(continued)

Class	Brand Names	Cost of a Month's Starting Dose	Manufacturer*
Thiazolidinediones	Actos	$94	Takeda/Lilly
	Avandia	$78	GlaxoSmithKline
Others	Glucophage	$38	Bristol-Myers Squibb
	Glucovance	$39	Bristol-Myers Squibb
	Prandin	$74	Novo Nordisk

*See appendix B for the phone numbers of the manufacturers.

Generic Substitution

The following diabetes drugs are available as generics. If you are prescribed the brand name, ask your pharmacist to call your doctor to request the generic brand. The difference in cost for a month's supply of the starting dose can be substantial.

Brand Name	Generic Name
DiaBeta	Glyburide
Diabinese	Chlopropamide
Glucophage	Metformin
Glucotrol	Glipizide
Glynase	Glyburide

Pill Cutting

Many diabetes drugs are available as tablets in various strengths. The prices are usually the same for the different strengths, so if you are at a lower dose, ask your doctor to prescribe the higher dose and then split it. First ask for assistance from your pharmacist to make sure you are splitting the pill correctly. If you are, the savings can be substantial. and you can actually cut your cost in half.

Drug Company Assistance Programs

The table on page 175 shows the various drugs for diabetes and their manufacturers. If you have been prescribed any of these products and you cannot afford them, call the manufacturer (see appendix B) and explain your situation. You might end up with free drugs. If a manufacturer is not listed, then that manufacturer does not have an assistance program at this time.

Other Strategies to Reduce Medication Costs

Revisit chapters 4 and 5 for strategies like samples, mail order, discount programs, and state government programs. Use as many as you can. The more programs you use, the more savings you will achieve.

Indirect Costs

Indirect costs are costs incurred as a result of the disease preventing the individual from being a more productive member of society. These indirect costs were estimated to total $54 billion in 1997 and are expected to be significantly higher today. These costs come from:

- Time lost from work due to disability and sick days
- Premature retirement
- Premature death

Indirect costs are higher than direct costs, hence society as a whole suffers a significant burden when an individual is stricken with diabetes.

If you have diabetes, you may be worried about the effect it might have on your job. What if it causes you to require more sick days than normal? What happens if you have to ask for time to check your glucose or inject insulin? Would you be considered less of an asset? Do you have a disability for which you could be fired? The last question actually provides us the answer. Technically, the government has classified people who have diabetes as having a disability and that gives them protection under the Americans with Disability Act (ADA). Under this law, an employer who employs 15 or more people cannot discriminate against any individual who has a disability. This protection covers hiring, firing, promotion, pay, and other benefits. However, the ADA covers only private employers. The Rehabilitation Act of 1973 covers government employees, and any employer who receives federal money is prohibited from discriminating against people with disabilities.

The Family and Medical Leave Act of 1993 allows you to take up to 12 weeks of unpaid leave each year to care for yourself or a family member with a serious illness. If the complication of your diabetes requires time off to deal with it, this law would ensure that you do not lose your job.

The important thing to remember about your diabetes and your job is not to give the employer reasons to believe that your disease is affecting your performance. This requires that you plan ahead. Pay attention to special circumstances that could affect your diabetes care routine. This includes traveling, working odd hours, or attending long meetings.

Intangible Costs

There are other costs associated with diabetes that are difficult to attach numbers to. These are called intangible or psychological costs and actually have a great effect on the life of the patient and the family. These come from such items as pain, anxiety, stress, family members adjusting to the patient's illness, and the effect of the premature death of the patient on the ones left behind.

Family

There are three main areas in which an individual's diabetes can affect the relationship with family members and create concerns:

- Lifestyle changes
- Dealing with stress and depression related to having diabetes
- Sexual relationships

Lifestyle Changes

Lifestyle changes involve diet and exercise. People who have diabetes might have to change the way they have been eating all their lives to help keep the disease under control. This could mean having two sets of meals, one for the person with diabetes and one for everybody else. If that happens, the cost of feeding the family can increase. This does not have to be the case. If the changes are accomplished in a gradual fashion, the whole family can adjust to it and no special diets need be prepared for anybody.

The other main lifestyle change is to exercise regularly. As stated in chapter 2, this does not have to involve any costs. Getting family members involved in activities designed to increase your activity level can actually make it more fun and more sustainable.

Dealing with Stress and Depression

Having diabetes can create a lot of stress for the patient as well as for loved ones. Family members might have to adjust their schedules to better meet the needs of someone with diabetes, such as in dealing with insulin shots, waiting for the person to check glucose levels, or avoiding certain activities and foods that other members want because they think it will affect their blood sugar. There is also the fear of the unknown, such as wondering what this might mean for the future of the family. Would it mean job loss, not having children, or making changes in the house to accommodate an advanced diabetic with complications?

People who have diabetes are also two to four times more likely to be depressed than those who do not have diabetes. This can be stressful for other family members who might not know how to react to the depression. Some strategies to deal with these issues include:

- Educating the whole family about diabetes
- Joining support groups of other diabetics
- Seeking counseling if needed
- Openly discussing your feelings
- Planning for emergencies, both medically and financially

Sexual Relationships

Diabetes can affect the sex lives of both men and women. This in turn can put a strain on the relationship and create other unforeseen consequences. This could affect communication between partners and deprive the relationship of quality time.

For women diabetes can lead to:

- Increased yeast infections
- Reduced vaginal lubrication
- Reduced sensitivity in the genitals
- Poor bladder control
- Reduced sexual desire
- Limited mobility arising from loss of a limb

In men, diabetes can lead to impotence or erection problems. While a large number of men with diabetes, especially those over age 50, suffer from impotence, it is important to distinguish between impotence caused by the diabetes and impotence caused by psychological factors. One of the ways to distinguish this is to see if you have erections in your sleep. If you do, then your impotence is most probably psychological. This would have to be treated by dealing with the psychological events causing this, and you might have to see a mental health professional. Your primary care doctor can treat the impotence caused by diabetes, with either devices or medications.

To minimize the effect of diabetes on the sex life of the patient and the partner:

- Maintain good blood glucose control.
- Talk openly about your sex life with each other.
- Discuss ways to put more spark into your sex life.
- Make time away from work and your kids to spend with each other.

Alternative Remedies

According to the National Institute of Diabetes and Digestive and Kidney Diseases (NIDDK), the government agency at the forefront of diabetes research, the following alternative therapies have been used to help individuals manage their diabetes: acupuncture, biofeedback, guided imagery, and vitamins and mineral supplements.

Acupuncture

Acupuncture helps in reducing the pain caused by damaged nerves in diabetic patients. Chronic pain is experienced by a lot of diabetics. The use of acupuncture can be less expensive than the management of the pain through conventional therapy, especially for those not covered by insurance.

Biofeedback

Biofeedback is a powerful relaxation technique that has been used to help individuals become more aware of the body's response to pain and other health signals. This allows people to better manage and deal with such signals as pain and to better deal with stress.

Guided Imagery

This is also a relaxation technique. In this method, the individual is asked to focus on a peaceful and pleasant image such as a beautiful beach. It is felt that the more the individual can focus on the positive image and direct mental energies away from the diseased body, the better the body can deal with the disease.

Vitamins and Minerals

The following vitamins and minerals may help in the treatment of diabetes:

Chromium. Chromium has been extensively studied for diabetes, and there are reports that it can improve diabetes control. The thought is that chromium can help insulin work better.

Magnesium. If your body lacks magnesium, blood glucose control especially in type 2 diabetes gets worse. It is believed that the pancreas needs magnesium to effectively release insulin and also that magnesium is needed to reduce insulin resistance and hence increase its efficiency. Lack of magnesium can lead to greater complications in a diabetic.

Vanadium. One recent study showed that when diabetics were given vanadium, a compound found in very tiny amounts in plants and animals, they developed an increase in insulin sensitivity and were able to reduce their insulin requirements.

As with all alternative therapies, be sure to inform your doctor before starting any alternative therapy and inform your doctor if you are taking any herbs or supplements, especially if you are taking prescription medications.

Resources

American Association of
  Diabetes Educators
(800) 338-3633
www.aadenet.org

American Diabetes Association
(800) 342-2383
www.diabetes.org

American Dietetic Association
(800) 877-1600
www.eatright.org

Juvenile Diabetes Research
  Foundation
(800) 223-1138
www.jdrf.org

National Diabetes Information
  Clearing House
(301) 654-3327
www.niddk.org

CHAPTER 15

Heart Disease

Heart disease is the number one killer of individuals. Each year more than one and a half million people have heart attacks and half a million die from heart disease. The risk factors that can contribute to heart disease include:

- High blood pressure
- Cigarette smoking
- Diabetes
- High cholesterol
- Excessive stress
- Physical inactivity

A heart attack occurs when one or more of the major vessels that supply the heart with blood become obstructed and blood does not reach that part of the heart. Damage or death occurs to that part of the heart and the person experiences the symptoms of a heart attack. If it is severe enough the individual might collapse and die before help arrives.

Heart Attack Warning Signs

Some heart attacks are sudden and intense. However, most heart attacks start slowly, with mild pain or discomfort. Often people affected aren't sure what's wrong and wait too long before getting help. The following are signs that can mean a heart attack is happening:

- *Chest discomfort.* Most heart attacks involve discomfort in the center of the chest that lasts more than a few minutes, or that goes away and comes back. It can feel like uncomfortable pressure, squeezing, fullness, or pain.

- *Discomfort in other areas of the upper body.* Symptoms can include pain or discomfort in one or both arms, the back, neck, jaw, or abdomen.
- *Shortness of breath.* This feeling often accompanies chest discomfort, but it can also occur before the chest discomfort.
- *Other signs.* These may include a cold sweat, nausea, or lightheadedness.

If you or someone you're with has chest discomfort, especially with one or more of the other signs, don't wait longer than a few minutes (no more than five) before calling for help.

Calling 911 is usually the fastest way to get lifesaving treatment. Emergency medical services staff can begin treatment when they arrive—up to an hour sooner than if someone gets to the hospital by car. The staff is also trained to revive someone whose heart has stopped. You'll also get treated faster in the hospital if you come by ambulance.

If you can't access the emergency medical services (EMS) through calling 911, have someone drive you to the hospital right away. If you're the one having symptoms, don't drive yourself unless you have absolutely no other option. Some doctors advise chewing on an aspirin while waiting for the ambulance to arrive. At the hospital, the goal is to restore blood to the damaged areas and get the heart back to normal as much as is possible. When the patient is discharged, the goal is to address the underlying cause of the heart attack and to prescribe a lifestyle that will maintain a healthy heart.

Several damages to the heart can eventually lead to heart failure, requiring a heart transplant, or if none is found, then an early death.

In this chapter, we will focus on two disease states that are well-known risk factors for causing heart attacks: high blood pressure, also known as hypertension, and high blood cholesterol.

High Blood Pressure

The Centers for Disease Control and Prevention estimate that more than 50 million North Americans age six and older have high blood pressure. This means that about 25 percent of all adult North Americans have high blood pressure. Since untreated high blood pressure causes heart attacks and strokes, controlling high blood pressure is crucial. High blood pressure has no symptoms, which makes it a serious problem to control.

What Is High Blood Pressure?

Blood pressure is the measure of the force of blood as it travels through the blood vessels. The arteries are the vessels that bring blood to the organs. As they get close to the organs, their walls contract and expand, which changes the resistance to blood flow. Contraction increases the resistance, and reduces blood flow. This increases blood pressure and causes the heart to work harder. Blood pressure is needed to keep blood flowing and the changes in blood pressure ensure that the different parts of the body get the amount of blood needed to keep them functioning. For example, when you exercise, your muscles need more blood, so the small arteries in the muscles relax to let more blood flow into the muscles.

Blood pressure measurement has two readings, a systolic blood pressure and a diastolic blood pressure. The systolic pressure is the force of blood flow when the heart beats. The diastolic pressure is the pressure between heartbeats while the heart is at rest. So when you get a blood pressure reading of 120/80, the first number (120) represents the systolic reading and the second number (80) is the diastolic blood pressure.

Blood pressure increases with age, and there is a wide variation of what is considered normal. Doctors usually begin worrying when the reading is higher than 140/90 mm Hg. Usually your doctor will take several readings before a diagnosis of high blood pressure is made. He or she might even ask you to measure your blood pressure at home due to the fact that many people become very nervous when they see their doctor and the readings are not accurate. This phenomenon is called white coat hypertension, for the white coats that doctors wear.

Symptoms

High blood pressure is your classic "silent killer" since there are no symptoms. For many individuals, the first sign that they have high blood pressure is when they have a heart attack or stroke, and on examination it is revealed that their blood pressure has been high for years.

Types

There are two types of high blood pressure: primary or essential hypertension and secondary hypertension.

Primary or Essential Hypertension

Approximately 90–95 percent of all cases of hypertension are primary hypertension. Nobody knows what causes primary hypertension.

Secondary Hypertension

Secondary hypertension is caused by an underlying disorder. Some of the conditions that can cause blood pressure to increase are:

- Brain tumors
- Hypercalcemia, a condition of excessive calcium
- Disease of the adrenal glands
- Kidney disease
- Thyroid disease
- Sleep disturbances
- Disease of the aorta, the biggest artery

In order to treat the hypertension, the disease that caused it must be diagnosed and treated.

Complications

High blood pressure is not often listed as the cause of death. The danger of high blood pressure is that it is causes so many complications that then result in something catastrophic. The main conditions that high blood pressure can lead to are:

- Heart attacks (discussed earlier)
- Heart failure
- Blood vessel damage
- Strokes
- Kidney damage

Heart Failure

When your blood pressure stays high, the heart has to work harder to push blood through the blood vessels. What happens if you have to lift heavy loads often? You develop bigger muscles. The heart, being a muscle, becomes thicker to continue working against this increased load. Eventually, however, the heart just can't keep up anymore and fails.

Blood Vessel Damage

Sustained increase in blood pressure results in the weakening of the arteries. The main artery, the aorta, can eventually become weak enough in certain spots to develop what is known as an aneurysm. This is when a bulge occurs on the artery walls from the weakening of the wall. This weakened area can eventually burst open, leading to internal bleeding and death.

Strokes

Just as we described with the heart, the blood vessels that supply the brain with blood can become blocked or clamp down. When this happens, the part of the brain that loses blood supply will die. With the heart, when a part dies, the result is felt in the heart itself. With the brain, if an area dies, the part of the body that the brain controls becomes affected. So, for example, if the part of the brain that controls leg movements is destroyed, the stroke victim will become paralyzed. A stroke can also lead outright to death.

Kidney Damage

There are millions of little cups in the kidney called glomeruli. It is in these cups that the kidney cleans the blood, getting rid of wastes and also helping to regulate the amount of water in the body. Sustained high blood pressure destroys these cups. As more and more of these cups are destroyed, the kidney progressively loses its ability to clean the blood and regulate the water content. The patient eventually has to have dialysis, where a machine takes over the functions of the kidney, or the patient gets a new kidney.

Prevention

Because we do not know why most cases of high blood pressure occur, designing prevention programs is very difficult. However, there are risk factors that contribute to high blood pressure. The more you know about them, the more likely you are to get your blood pressure checked on a regular basis.

The controllable risk factors include:

- Obesity or excess weight
- Eating too much salt
- Alcohol
- Lack of exercise
- Stress

The following factors cannot be controlled:

- *Race.* African Americans have higher rates of high blood pressure than white Americans.
- *Heredity.* High blood pressure tends to run in families.
- *Age.* In general, the older you get, the greater your chance of developing high blood pressure.

Managing the Cost

High blood pressure as a disease is not what we observe, hence it is difficult to accurately figure out its direct costs. However, since it can lead to heart disease and strokes, it is important to prevent or control it.

According to the American Heart Association, the cost of managing heart disease and stroke was $326.6 billion in the United States in 2000.

Direct costs incurred in trying to treat the disease include:

- Physician visits and tests
- Medications
- Hospitalization

Physician Visits and Tests

You need to have your blood pressure tested on a regular basis if you are at risk, and annually even if you are not. Doctors routinely do blood pressure tests whenever you visit them. The cost for this visit is usually your copay, which will range from $5 to $20 for most HMO plans. If you have indemnity insurance, you will usually pay 20 percent of the doctor's fees and the plan pays for 80 percent of the fees that are deemed allowable.

In most HMO plans, you are allowed the copay only if you see your primary care physician. If you decide to see a physician outside the plan's network or visit a specialist without getting a referral from your primary care physician, your plan would most likely make you pay nearly all the cost of that visit. Primary care physicians can easily diagnose high blood pressure. So to be cost-wise, schedule an appointment with your primary care physician instead of a specialist.

After you visit your physician and you are diagnosed with high blood pressure, it is important to realize that this is a lifelong problem, one that can lead to serious consequences if not kept under control. Your blood pressure must be monitored, and if you are given medicine to control it, you might have to come back several times to make sure it is working. To reduce the number of physician visits, it is important to ask your doctor as many questions as you can during that initial visit to understand what you need to do to control the disease and what types of unusual things might occur when you start therapy. You must also provide the doctor with as much information as you can about your lifestyle because this might help the doctor tailor a program for you and also let you know what you need to modify.

Make sure these topics are part of your conversation with your doctor:

- Your medical history: whether you have or had any other diseases
- Your family history of diseases including heart disease, strokes, and diabetes
- Your current lifestyle: eating, drinking, smoking, drug use
- Exercise history
- If you are taking any medications
- Side effects you might experience with your medications
- Whether you should you do home monitoring

Your doctor may also take X rays, EKGs, and other tests to determine how much damage the high blood pressure has done to your body.

Never be shy about calling your doctor if you have questions about your disease state or your treatment. A lot of visits can be saved by clearly following your doctor's advice and calling with questions about things you might be experiencing.

If You Do Not Have Insurance

If you do not have health insurance, there are still ways to get tested. Many hospitals and community centers offer routine blood pressure screenings. Even many local drug stores have blood pressure machines that you can use for a nominal fee, or you can call advocacy groups, such as the American Heart Association (see the end of this chapter for names and numbers), and ask for centers in your area where you can get tested for free. Health fairs almost always provide tests for blood pressure.

Check to see if there are any federally funded clinics in the area. These clinics provide services for reduced fees and accept payments on a sliding scale based on income. If these are not available, the last alternative is to call around for physicians and let them know that you think you might have high blood pressure and that you need to be tested. Remember to call only primary care physicians (internists or family doctors) and not specialists who are more expensive.

Blood pressure readings are the only way to monitor control. You can get it done at your doctor's office or do it at home. You might ask the doctor's nurse to do it. This will save you money, and you won't have to pay for a doctor's visit. Of course, if the blood pressure reading is too high or too low, you should see the doctor.

If you suffer from "white coat hypertension" (see page 184), the reading at your doctor's office might not reflect your true reading. The American Society of Hypertension now advises monitoring your blood pressure at home. When you first get a home blood pressure machine, take it to your doctor to verify its accuracy. Once that is accomplished, use the machine at home to monitor your blood pressure frequently. Keep a record of the readings and take the results with you when you visit your doctor.

Unfortunately, home blood pressure monitors are not covered by insurance companies despite pleas by medical organizations for them to do so. If you have high blood pressure though, you should buy one. There are a wide variety of machines with prices that range from as low as $15. Shop around for prices. The styles also vary, from manual to automatic, from digital to analogue, from arm to wrist and even finger monitors. No matter which type you get, as stated earlier, be sure to have your doctor verify that it is accurate.

Medications

If diet and exercise fail to control your blood pressure, the next step is to add medications. You should always start with one medication, known as monotherapy. This cuts down on chances of side effects and also reduces your medication costs. If one drug fails to achieve control, another might have to be added.

The following table shows the different classes and drugs used to manage high blood pressure, as well as the manufacturer of the drug.

Class	Brand Names	Cost of a Month's Starting Dose	Manufacturer*
Angiotensin-converting enzyme (ACE) inhibitors	Accupril	$30	Pfizer
	Altace	$32	Monarch
	Capoten	$45	Bristol-Myers Squibb
	Lotensin	$28	Novartis
	Monopril	$28	Bristol-Myers Squibb
	Prinivil	$29	Merck
	Vasotec	$30	Merck
Angiotensin receptor antagonist	Atacand	$41	AstraZeneca
	Avapro	$41	Bristol-Myers Squibb
	Cozaar	$41	Merck
	Diovan	$42	Novartis
	Micardis	$42	Boehringer Ingelheim
Beta blockers	Blocadren	$32	Merck
	Corgard	$42	Bristol-Myers Squibb
	Inderal-LA	$32	Wyeth
	Kerlone	$30	Pharmacia
	Levatol	$43	Schwarz
	Lopressor	$29	Novartis
	Normodyne	$39	Schering
	Sectral	$50	Wyeth
	Ternomin	$28	AstraZeneca
	Toprol XL	$20	AstraZeneca
	Visken	$72	Novartis
	Zebeta	$48	Lederle
Diuretics	Aldactone	$29	Pharmacia
	Demadex	$20	Roche
	Diuril	$12	Merck
	Edecrin	$15	Merck
	Lasix	$15	Aventis
	Lozol	$30	Aventis
	Midamor	$16	Merck
	Mykrox	$34	Celltech
	Zaroxolyn	$31	Celltech

Class	Brand Names	Cost of a Month's Starting Dose	Manufacturer*
Calcium	Adalat CC	$38	Bayer
channel	Calan SR	$38	Pharmacia
blockers	Cardene SR	$45	Roche
	Cardizem CD	$45	Biovail
	Corvera-HS	$40	Pharmacia
	Norvasc	$40	Pfizer
	Plendil	$33	Merck
	Procardia XL	$40	Pfizer
	Sular	$34	AstraZeneca
	Verelan PM	$42	Schwarz
Alpha	Aldomet	$23	Merck
adrenergic	Catapress TT	$38	Boehringer Ingelheim
blockers	Cardura	$33	Pfizer
	Hytrin	$55	Abbott
	Minipress	$30	Pfizer
	Tenex	$40	Robins
	Wytensin	$54	Wyeth
Direct vasodilators	Loniten	$47	Pharmacia

*See appendix B for the phone numbers of the manufacturers.

Let's examine some of the techniques that can be used to achieve savings on drugs for high blood pressure.

Brand-Name Substitution

As you can see from the table, there are many drugs for high blood pressure. Prices for a month's supply vary considerably, from about $12 to more than $70. High blood pressure is probably the disease with the greatest number of drugs approved to manage it. There are also many classes of drugs for the treatment of high blood pressure. So no matter what class of drugs your doctor decides to start you on, there are choices. Discuss with your doctor about beginning with a less expensive one unless there is a reason not to. Many patients with high blood pressure have to take more than one medication for their condition. Even if this is the case, your doctor has many to choose from.

Generic Substitution

As shown in the following table, many blood pressure medications are available as generics. If you are prescribed the brand name, ask your pharmacist to call your doctor to request the generic brand. The difference in cost for a month's supply of the starting dose can be substantial.

Brand Name	Generic Name
Adalat CC	Nifedipine
Aldactone	Spironolactone
Aldomet	Methyldopa
Blocadren	Timolol
Calan SR	Verapamil
Capoten	Captopril
Cardene SR	Nicardipine
Cardizem CD	Diltiazem
Cardura	Doxazosine
Catapress TT	Clonidine
Corgard	Nadolol
Corvera HS	Verapamil
Diuril	Chlorothiaxide
Hytrin	Terazosin
Inderal—LA	Propranolol
Lasix	Furosemide
Loniten	Minoxidil
Lopressor	Metoprolol
Lotensin	Benazepril
Lozol	Indapamide
Midamor	Amiloride
Minipress	Prazosin
Mykrox	Metolazone
Normodyne	Labetolol
Prinivil	Lisinopril
Procardia XL	Nifedipine
Sectral	Acebutolol

Brand Name	Generic Name
Tenex	Guanfacine
Tenormin	Atenolol
Toprol XL	Matoprolol
Vasotec	Enalapril
Verelan	Verapamil
Visken	Pindolol
Wytensin	Guanabenz
Zaroxolyn	Metolazone
Zebeta	Bisoprolol

Drug Company Assistance Programs

Appendix B lists the phone numbers of the various manufacturers of blood pressure medications. If a manufacturer is not listed then that drug is not available for the patient assistance program. If you have been prescribed any of the drugs for high blood pressure and you cannot afford it, call the manufacturer and explain your situation. If you need help in navigating the process, call one of the companies listed in chapter 5 for assistance.

Other Strategies to Reduce Medication Costs

Revisit chapters 4 and 5 for strategies like samples, mail order, discount programs, and state government programs. Use as many as you can. The more programs you use, the more savings you will achieve.

Hospitalization

High blood pressure can result in hospitalizations from the conditions that were described in the section on complications: heart attacks, heart failure, blood vessel damage, stroke, and kidney failure. Another condition that can result in hospitalization from high blood pressure is known as hypertensive emergency. This occurs when your blood pressure gets so high that it needs to be brought down quickly to avoid serious damage to organs or to prevent death. Usually you do not feel any symptoms with high blood pressure. Sometimes, though, when you are in a hypertensive emergency, you might feel such symptoms as headache, blurred vision, chest pain, and shortness of breath. It is a good idea to check your blood pressure if you feel these symptoms. That is why it is advisable to have a blood pressure monitor at home.

If your blood pressure is too high, usually above 180/110, it needs to be brought down immediately. You should be taken to the emergency room, where doctors will be able to lower it.

Hospitalizations for cardiovascular diseases and strokes are some of the most expensive hospital stays because they usually involve various procedures, some of which can be very complex. Also, because these events can come on suddenly, there is little chance for preparations. An individual with high blood pressure that is not adequately controlled must realize that there is a good chance of ending up in the hospital from any of the complications from high blood pressure—if the person doesn't die first. It has been clearly established that if high blood pressure is controlled, the chances of developing any of the complications drops significantly.

What this means is that if you have high blood pressure, do everything you can to control it. If you are not controlling it, then make all the necessary financial and legal arrangements in case you end up in the hospital. This means checking to make sure you have health insurance and have done the necessary estate planning.

If You Do Not Have Insurance

If you don't have insurance, it is essential to control your blood pressure. Hospital stays can be very expensive. Dying isn't cheap either because of the burden left behind. Chapter 7 describes what you should do to manage hospital bills if you do not have insurance, but most people can avoid hospitalization from the complications of high blood pressure if they can keep it under control.

When high blood pressure leads to strokes, it can be devastating. Many times, the individual doesn't die immediately but becomes paralyzed. Many of these patients never fully recover. Stroke victims are often discharged from the hospital not to return home, but to go to nursing homes or rehabilitation facilities. These facilities might not be covered by your regular health insurance. You need long-term care or some other form of insurance to cover these services.

Indirect Costs

Indirect costs are costs incurred as a result of the disease preventing the individual from being a more productive member of society. The indirect costs include:

- Time lost from work due to disability and sick days
- Premature retirement
- Premature death

High blood pressure by itself does not qualify someone as being disabled; hence the person cannot get the protections that the Americans with Disability Act (ADA) gives to individuals in the workplace. However, if as a result of high blood pressure you end up with a heart attack, stroke, or kidney damage, you might become disabled and thus will get the protections given by the ADA. These protections include having your employer make reasonable accommodations to allow you to perform the essential features of your job, as well as enjoying all the benefits that the other workers enjoy.

If you come down with a disease because of your high blood pressure, you will also get protection from the Family and Medical Leave Act, which allows you to take up to 12 weeks of unpaid leave each year to care for yourself or a family member with a serious illness.

Intangible Costs

Family

There are two main areas in which an individual's high blood pressure can affect the relationship with family members and create concerns: lifestyle changes and sexual relationships.

Lifestyle Changes

Lifestyle changes involve diet and exercise. A person with high blood pressure might have to change the eating habits of a lifetime to help keep the disease under control. This could mean eating foods that are low in fat and have less salt. The other main lifestyle change is to exercise regularly. As stated previously, this does not have to involve any costs. Getting family members involved in activities designed to increase your activity level can actually make it more fun and more sustainable. Any changes in one's lifestyle might be disruptive in relationships. The key here is to communicate and let the other members understand the importance of your lifestyle changes. Be sensitive to the others' needs and take them into account as you make these changes.

Sexual Relationships

Since the act of sexual relations can cause your blood pressure to go up, some people might be reluctant or even afraid to have sex. You should talk to your doctor about this. Also, in men, some of the drugs used to treat high blood pressure can cause impotence or erection problems. While a large number of men with high blood pressure, especially those over age 50, suffer from impotence, it is important to distinguish between impotence caused by the high blood pressure and that caused by the drugs used to treat it and psychological factors. One of the ways to distinguish this is to see if you have erections in your sleep. If you do, then your impotence is most probably psychological. This would have to be treated by dealing with the psychological events causing this and you might have to see a mental health professional. Your primary care doctor can treat the impotence caused by high blood pressure, with either devices or medications.

Complementary and Alternative Therapies

DASH

There is a complementary therapy for high blood pressure that involves using a type of diet. It can be used effectively with medications or by itself to reduce blood pressure. It is known as the DASH diet, which stands for Dietary Approaches to Stop Hypertension. DASH began as a clinical study that examined the effect on blood pressure of various diet plans. It compared the effect on blood pressure of three meal plans: a regular American diet, a diet similar to a regular American meal but higher in fruits and vegetables, and the DASH plan, which was a diet low in saturated fat, total fat, and cholesterol and rich in fruits, vegetables, and low-fat dairy. The DASH diet also included whole grains, poultry, fish, and nuts and reduced the amounts of red meats, sweets, and sugared beverages.

The result was dramatic. The DASH diet reduced blood pressure to levels seen with the use of medications. The effect was observed as early as two weeks after the participants went on the plan. A second study, called DASH-Sodium, showed that on the DASH plan, if salt was reduced the blood pressure could be reduced even more.

Based on these results, individuals with high blood pressure are advised to modify their diet to that used in DASH. To accomplish this with as little disruption as possible, use the box on the following page as your guide.

As a word of caution, do not stop taking your medications when you get on the plan. Discuss with your doctor what you are doing and he or she might adjust your medications if needed.

Other Complementary Therapies

A number of other therapies have been shown to be beneficial in reducing blood pressure. They include:

Stress management. Stress has been shown to increase the hormones in our bodies that increase blood pressure. Stress management techniques such as relaxation, meditation, and biofeedback can reduce blood pressure.

Potassium supplements. Individuals who consume low amounts of potassium have higher blood pressure. Increasing potassium levels, either through supplements or foods such as bananas, can reduce blood pressure, especially in populations like African Americans whose diets might be low in potassium.

Fish oil supplements. Fish oil, known as omega-3 polyunsaturated fatty acid (n-3 PUFA), can be found as supplements or obtained from fatty fishes like salmon. It has been shown that moderate to high doses of n-3 PUFA can reduce blood pressures in patients whose blood pressures were not being treated.

High Blood Cholesterol

High blood cholesterol is one of the biggest risk factors for a heart attack. It is now estimated that 65 million North Americans should watch their diet to reduce their cholesterol levels and 36 million of those should actually be on cholesterol-lowering medications.

What Is Cholesterol?

The fats that are in your blood are called lipids. Cholesterol is one of the major lipids. It is a waxy substance produced by the liver and is also supplied in the diet through animal products such as meats, poultry, fish, and dairy products. You need cholesterol to live. It helps insulate nerves and make cell membranes, and is used for the production of some hormones. As our bodies are capable of making all the choles-

---

Getting Started on the DASH Meal Plan

It's easy to adopt the DASH eating plan. Here are some ways to get started:

Change gradually.

- If you now eat one or two vegetables a day, add a serving at lunch and another at dinner.
- If you don't eat fruit now or have only juice at breakfast, add a serving to your meals or have it as a snack.
- Gradually increase your use of fat-free and low-fat dairy products. For example, drink milk with lunch or dinner instead of soda, sugar-sweetened tea, or alcohol. Choose low-fat (1%) or fat-free (skim) dairy products to reduce your intake of saturated fat, total fat, cholesterol, and calories.
- Read food labels on margarines and salad dressings to choose those lowest in unsaturated fat. Some margarines are now trans-fat free.

Treat meat as one part of the whole meal, instead of the focus.

- Limit meat to 6 ounces a day (two servings); that's all that's needed. Three to four ounces is about the size of a deck of cards.
- If you now eat large portions of meat, cut back gradually by a half or a third at each meal.
- Include two or more vegetarian-style (meatless) meals each week.
- Increase servings of vegetables, rice, pasta, and dry beans in meals. Try casseroles and pasta, and stir-fry dishes, which have less meat and more vegetables, grains, and dry beans.

terol we need, we do not need to eat foods that contain cholesterol to keep up the level.

There are different types of cholesterol. The two most important for your cardiovascular health are: low-density lipoprotein (LDL) and high-density lipoprotein (HDL).

LDL is called the "bad cholesterol" because it is the main source of cholesterol build-up in the arteries that can eventually lead to blockage. HDL is the "good cholesterol" because it prevents cholesterol from building up in the arteries.

When your cholesterol levels are checked, your doctor will look at the amount of LDL, HDL, and the total cholesterol levels (TCL). Another fat that is usually checked is triglyceride. The primary goal of therapy is to reduce the level of LDL and TCL. The following tables show how these cholesterols are categorized.

LDL Cholesterol Levels	Category
Less than 100 mg/dL	Optimal
100–129 mg/dL	Near optimal
130–159 mg/dL	Borderline high
160–189 mg/dL	High
190 mg/dL and above	Very high

Total Cholesterol Levels	Category
Less than 200 mg/dL	Desirable
200–239 mg/dL	Borderline high
240 mg/dL and above	High

The goals for HDL and triglyceride levels are HDL levels of 60 mg/dL and above and triglycerides of less than 200 mg/dL.

Symptoms

High cholesterol itself has no symptoms and that makes it even more dangerous. Many individuals have high cholesterol and do not know it. The only way to find out if you have high cholesterol is to get your blood examined. A routine physical examination is vital when it comes to managing your cholesterol to decrease your chances of having a heart attack or stroke.

Complications

As you can imagine, any time you prevent blood flow to an area of the body that area will get damaged. By building up in the arteries and choking off blood supply, high cholesterol can in essence destroy any part of our bodies. The two main organs that get affected are the heart and the brain. When cholesterol builds up and blocks blood vessels supplying blood to parts of the heart or brain we end up with a heart attack or a stroke, respectively.

Prevention

What we do and what we eat can control the cholesterol level in our blood. Things to avoid because they increase cholesterol include:

- Saturated fats and cholesterol in foods. Reduce the intake of animal fats and oils that contain saturated fats, such as liver, egg yolks, and full-fat dairy products.
- Lack of exercise. If you stay inactive, you reduce your body's ability to reduce fats naturally.
- Being overweight. Obesity has been shown to be related to increased cholesterol levels.
- Smoking. It has been shown to increase LDL and decrease HDL, so stop smoking.

You can lower your LDL through:

- Exercise. This has been shown not only to decrease LDL, but also to also increase HDL, so start exercising.
- Diet. It is not just what you don't eat but also what you eat. Certain oils like olive oil and fish oil from fishes like salmon have been shown to affect our blood cholesterol favorably. Also, foods that are good sources of soluble fiber like oats, fruits (oranges and pears), vegetables (brussels sprouts, carrots, and peas), and beans can all reduce cholesterol.

There are other things that can increase cholesterol levels, but that you have no control over. These include:

- Age. As you get older your cholesterol levels go up.
- Gender. Women, especially after menopause, experience increased cholesterol levels.

- Genetics. We inherit genes that determine how our bodies make and use cholesterol.

While we cannot control these things, if we are in any of these categories then we should do even more to manage the things we can do.

Managing the Cost

Like high blood pressure, high cholesterol itself is not what kills you. It does lead to heart attacks and strokes. This makes it hard to measure high cholesterol's direct costs. However, if you consider the number of hospitalizations and deaths from heart attacks, it is obvious that lowering cholesterol will save lives and money.

The direct costs incurred in trying to treat the disease include:

- Physician visits
- Medications
- Hospitalization

Physician Visits

As you get older, regular cholesterol tests should be part of your physical. Everyone age 20 and older should get a complete cholesterol check at least every five years, according to the latest guidelines. As you get older, you should get them more often. Your doctor can do a blood test and measure your cholesterol levels.

The cost for this visit is usually your copay, which will range from $5 to $20 for most HMO plans. If you have indemnity insurance, you will usually pay 20 percent of the doctor's fees.

After you visit your physician and you are diagnosed with high cholesterol, it is important to realize that this is a life-long problem, and one that can lead to serious consequences if not kept under control. Your cholesterol must be monitored, and you might be given medicine to control it. Many of the drugs can affect liver function, so you must see your doctor not only to check your cholesterol, but also to make sure the drug is not adversely affecting your liver. Make sure these topics are part of your conversation with your doctor:

- Your medical history (whether you have or had any other diseases)

- Your family history of diseases including heart disease, strokes, and diabetes
- Your current lifestyle (eating, drinking, smoking, and drug use)
- Your exercise history
- Whether you are taking any medications
- Side effects you might experience with your medications

If You Do Not Have Insurance

If you do not have health insurance, there are ways to still get tested. Many hospitals and community centers offer routine cholesterol screenings. Call advocacy groups, such as the American Heart Association (see "Resources" at the end of this chapter for names and numbers), and ask for centers in your area where you can get tested for free. Many health fairs provide free cholesterol screenings.

Also, check to see if there are any federally funded clinics in the area. These clinics provide services for reduced fees and accept payments on a sliding scale based on income. If these clinics are not available, the last alternative is to call around for physicians who might see you for reduced fees. Remember to call only primary care physicians (internists or family doctors) and not specialists, who are more expensive.

Blood tests are the only way to monitor control. You can get it done at your doctor's office, or do it at home with a home testing kit for cholesterol. If you are watching your cholesterol levels, you should think of getting one.

Medications

If diet and exercise fail to control your cholesterol, the next step is to add medications. A new class of drugs, known as statins, has had great success in lowering cholesterol. You may be familiar with many of these drugs, including Lipitor and Pravachol. Recently, Baychol was removed from the market by the FDA due to deaths caused by liver problems. This has caused many to worry about statins, but both the American Heart Association and the American College of Cardiology feel that the benefits outweigh the risks.

The following are the different classes of drugs to control cholesterol.

Class	Brand Names	Cost of a Month's Starting Dose	Manufacturer*
Statins	Lescol	$42	Novartis
	Lipitor	$55	Pfizer
	Mevacor	$62	Merck
	Pravachol	$64	Bristol-Myers Squibb
	Zocor	$102	Merck
Resins	Colestid	$54	Pharmacia
	Questran	$110	Bristol-Myers Squibb
Fibrates	Lopid	$78	Pfizer
	Tricor	$25	Abbott
Niacin	Niaspan	$35	Kos

*See appendix B for the phone numbers of the manufacturers.

Brand-Name Substitution

As the table shows, many drugs are available to manage high blood cholesterol and their prices can vary considerably, from a low of about $25 a month to at least $110 a month. While these prices might differ depending on where you shop, the differences in price among the drugs will probably be the same. So discuss with your doctor about starting with a less expensive drug in the same class, unless there is a reason not to.

Generic Substitution

The following drugs are available as generics. If you are prescribed the brand name, ask your pharmacist to call your doctor to request the generic. The difference in price between the generic and the brand name can be substantial.

Brand Name	Generic Name
Colestid	Colestipol
Lopid	Gemfibrozil
Mavachor	Lovastatin

Brand Name	Generic Name
Niaspan	Nicotinic acid
Questran	Cholestyramine
Tricor	Fenofibrate

Drug Company Assistance Programs

Appendix B gives the phone numbers of the various manufacturers. If a company is not listed, then as of this writing that company does not provide a patient assistance program. If you have been prescribed any of these products and you cannot afford them, call the number and explain your situation. If you need help in navigating the process, call one of the companies listed in chapter 5 for assistance.

Other Strategies to Reduce Medication Costs

Revisit chapters 4 and 5 for other strategies like samples, mail order, discount programs, and state government programs. Use as many as you can. The more programs you use, the more savings you will achieve.

Hospitalization

The issues related to hospitalization are the same as those with high blood pressure. You end up in the hospital because of the complications: heart attack or stroke. You might be fortunate if due to an examination or mild chest pain, it is discovered that one or more arteries are about to become blocked. In this case you will be admitted and the blockage will be cleared. Chest pain from reduced blood flow to the heart is known as angina and it is a sign that things might get worse.

A number of procedures are used to clear clogged arteries. The most common one is known as percutaneous transluminal cardiac angioplasty (PTCA). In this procedure a tube is inserted in a blood vessel and directed to the heart area where the blockage is and the blockage is removed. This requires considerable skill and is a very expensive procedure. After the blockage is dealt with, things are done to prevent it from coming back. This includes putting little rings in the area to keep it open, as well as using medications.

Procedures to deal with diseases of the heart—from angioplasty to open-heart surgery to a bypass, where a vein is used to actually go around the blockage, to a heart transplant—are some of the most expensive procedures done in the hospital. Yet admissions for cardio-vascular diseases still remain one of the top reasons for all hospitalizations.

In chapter 7, we discussed what to do if you are to be hospitalized. Unfortunately, in an emergency, as with a heart attack, you might not have time to plan these things. So if you have any of the risk factors for cardiovascular diseases, make sure your insurance policy is up to date; otherwise, if you end up in the hospital, it will cost you significant money.

If You Do Not Have Insurance

If you do not have insurance, pay careful attention to the strategies for what to do if you need to be hospitalized (see chapter 7). If you find yourself in an urgent situation, as opposed to an emergency, remember that public hospitals are the least expensive and specialist hospitals the most expensive. Also, some facilities can do some angioplasties on an outpatient basis. This will be less expensive that getting it done in an inpatient setting.

When it comes to heart procedures, it is important to remember that studies have shown that hospitals that perform high volumes of these procedures have better success rates than hospitals that do not. So check the experience of the hospital, as well as the experience of the person who will be performing the procedure. To any extent that you can, ask for references. If a high-volume hospital is expensive, you may still choose to get the procedure done there and arrange for a pay-ment plan with the hospital. No hospital will turn you away if you make a good-faith effort to honor your financial obligation.

Indirect Costs

The indirect costs related to high cholesterol come from lost produc-tivity arising from being hit by a heart attack or stroke. Many of the deaths from heart attacks are to individuals who are still in the prime of their lives. Such premature deaths not only deprive the family members of the person's income, but society suffers from not having the individ-ual contribute to the economy.

In terms of workplace protections, having high cholesterol does not make one disabled and hence the Americans with Disability Act

(ADA) does not protect an individual whose only symptom is high cholesterol. However, if high cholesterol leads to a heart attack or stroke and this creates a disability, you might be protected. You will, at this time, also have the protection of the Family and Medical Leave Act, which gives employees up to 12 weeks of unpaid leave to take care of themselves or a loved one with a medical condition.

Intangible Costs

There are other costs associated with high cholesterol. These intangible costs have a great effect on the life of the patient and the family. These come from such items as pain, anxiety, and stress. The most serious result of uncontrolled high cholesterol for family members is the premature death of the individual. When a heart attack cuts short the life of someone, especially when the person is still young, the effect can be devastating to family and friends.

Other Areas of Concern

Lifestyle Changes

Lifestyle changes may involve diet and exercise. A person with high cholesterol might have to change lifelong eating habits to help keep the disease under control. It is advisable to exercise regularly after seeking the advice of a physician and to eat low-fat meals. Quit smoking, and cut down on the intake of alcohol. These changes do not have to be expensive, and in some cases might even save you money. Getting family members involved in leading a healthy lifestyle is one way to ensure success.

Dealing with Stress

Having high cholesterol can create a lot of stress for the patient as well as for loved ones. There is the fear of the unknown, in other words, wondering what this might mean for the future of the family. The patient may worry about developing heart disease and about the side effects of medication, and may fear getting involved in situations that could increase his or her stress level. If you feel overwhelmed or helpless, or see these signs in your loved one, it is important to tell the doctor and get a referral to a mental health professional.

Sexual Relationships

High cholesterol can lead to erectile dysfunction because fat can deposit in the blood vessels that carry blood to the penis, decreasing its ability to maintain an erection. Also, some individuals who have heart problems might be concerned about engaging in sex, which can increase stress to the heart, for fear of having a heart attack. Some medications may also affect sexual desire. It is therefore important to keep an eye on how managing your cholesterol affects your sex life, and seek help if you need it. There are effective treatments for sexual difficulties that handle the medical as well as the psychological issues.

Complementary and Alternative Therapies

A number of supplements are being used to help manage high cholesterol and prevent cardiovascular diseases, thus reducing costs. Most of these work as antioxidants and prevent cholesterol from sticking to the blood vessels. These supplements include:

- Garlic, thought to lower cholesterol and prevent blood clots
- Ginger, also thought to lower cholesterol and prevent blood clots
- Folic acid, to reduce the level of homocysteine, a substance thought to make cholesterol more harmful
- Coenzyme Q10, thought to have antioxidant properties
- Vitamins B_6, B_{12}, C, and E, are all thought to prevent cholesterol from accumulating in the blood vessels
- Selenium, an antioxidant
- Chromium, shown to lower total cholesterol and to increase HDL
- Fish oil, to help prevent clots from forming where cholesterol is already building up

A lot of these supplements help not only in lowering cholesterol, but also in preventing clots from forming at the site of cholesterol buildup. It is estimated that about 90 percent of heart attacks and strokes are caused by blood clots forming at the site of cholesterol accumulation. It is therefore advisable to incorporate in our diets those nutrients and supplements that are known to fight blood clots at the same time that we work at reducing our cholesterol levels.

Resources

American Dietetic
Association
(800) 877-1600
www.eatright.org

American Heart
Association
(800) AHA-USA1
www.americanheart.org

Center for Disease Control
and Prevention (CDC)
(404) 639-3534
www.cdc.gov

National Heart, Lung, and
Blood Institute
(301) 496-4236
www.nhlbi.nih.gov

CHAPTER 16

HIV and AIDS

As of December 2000, about 780,000 cases of individuals with AIDS (Acquired Immune Deficiency Syndrome) have been reported in North America, and of these, about 450,000 have died. It is estimated that about 200,000 individuals are infected by HIV (Human Immunodeficiency Virus, the virus that causes AIDS) and are not aware of it. Luckily, cases of individuals with HIV infection peaked in 1993 and have been declining since then, although there is fear that HIV infection might be on the rise again. This decline in mortality has been brought about by education and widespread use of powerful drugs that can suppress the virus.

HIV disproportionately affects minorities, especially African Americans, and has become a leading killer of black males. AIDS affects seven times more African Americans and three times more Hispanics than whites.

What Are HIV and AIDS?

Cells in our blood called white blood cells fight germs like bacteria and viruses and keep us healthy. A lot of times, we are not even aware that we are infected by various bacteria and viruses as we go about our everyday lives, because our white blood cells are attacking and killing the bacteria. There are different types of white blood cells; the main one that fights off germs is called CD4+ T cell, or T4 cell. In a normal person, there are about 1,000 or more T4 cells per cubic millimeter of blood. When HIV enters the blood, it gets into the T4 cells and starts dividing rapidly. The virus then kills the cells as they release themselves. The infected individual might experience some flulike symptoms or have a rash. These symptoms disappear after a few days. The amount of virus in the blood—the viral load—then drops off and for the next month to even several years, the infected individual might have no symptoms.

After this quiet period, the viral load starts increasing and this increases the rate of destruction of the T4 cells. As the number of T4 cells decreases, the individual starts experiencing certain symptoms. From the initial infection to when these symptoms start occurring, the individual has HIV infection but is not considered to have AIDS. According to the Centers for Disease Control (CDC), the agency responsible for tracking diseases, AIDS occurs when the number of T4 cells falls below 200 cells per cubic millimeter and the patient can no longer fight infections. Other germs, in what are known as "opportunistic infections," start to attack the body.

Symptoms of HIV

When an individual is infected by the virus and is HIV-positive but does not yet have AIDS, he or she might experience a number of symptoms, including:

- Swollen glands in the neck, underarm, or groin area
- Lack of energy
- Weight loss
- Frequent fevers and sweats
- Persistent or frequent yeast infections (oral or vaginal)
- Persistent skin rashes or flaky skin
- Pelvic inflammatory disease in women that does not respond to treatment
- Short-term memory loss
- Frequent and severe herpes infections
- Shingles (a painful nerve disease)

These symptoms can occur with other diseases. However, if an individual experiences them for more than two weeks, the person should see a doctor, who would be able to rule out HIV infection as the cause.

Symptoms of AIDS

With AIDS, the body's immune system becomes so weak that bacteria or viruses that would normally not cause one to get sick now do so. These opportunistic infections are the hallmark of AIDS. They come from bacteria, viruses, fungi, parasites, and other germs. Opportunistic infections are what actually end up killing individuals with AIDS.

The symptoms of opportunistic infections include:

- Coughing and shortness of breath
- Seizures and lack of coordination
- Difficult or painful swallowing
- Mental symptoms such as confusion and forgetfulness
- Severe and persistent diarrhea
- Fever
- Vision loss
- Nausea, abdominal cramps, and vomiting
- Weight loss and extreme fatigue
- Severe headaches
- Coma

Individuals with AIDS are also prone to developing certain cancers, especially those that are caused by viruses. These include Kaposi's sarcoma, a skin cancer; cervical cancer; and lymphomas, which are cancers of the immune system.

Prevention of HIV Infection

HIV lives in the blood of an infected individual and can be transmitted to another individual when the blood, semen, vaginal fluid, or breast milk of the infected individual enters the body of a noninfected individual. The various means of transmission that have been identified are:

- Sexual intercourse, homosexual or heterosexual
- Sharing needles or other injection equipment
- Breastfeeding
- Childbirth
- Blood transfusion (now very rare)

It is estimated that almost half of all HIV infections are through homosexual contact between males, one quarter through injecting drugs, 10 percent through heterosexual contact, and only 1 percent through blood transfusion.

The areas of the body that are the usual entry points for the virus are the vagina, the mouth, the anus, the rectum, and through cuts and sores.

It is important to remember that the virus needs the blood to survive; hence it will not survive outside the body. This makes it impossible for the virus to be transmitted through casual contact. It also cannot go through unbroken skin or a latex barrier.

Preventing HIV infection involves taking steps to avoid the behaviors that put one at risk of having the virus transmitted. These are some of the things to keep in mind:

- Do not share needles or other injection equipment.
- Do not have unprotected sex, especially with multiple partners. Either abstain from having sex or use male latex condoms or female polyurethane condoms. Spermicides have not been shown to prevent transmission.
- Cover any cuts or sores if you have to come in contact with anyone who is HIV-infected.
- An HIV-infected mother should take medications to prevent transmission of the virus to the unborn child during birth or through breastfeeding.

High-Risk Groups

While anyone can contract AIDS if he or she practices risky behaviors, the following groups are more vulnerable:

- Homosexual or bisexual men who are sexually active
- Those who are present or past abusers of intravenous drugs
- Patients who have had transfusions of blood and blood products
- Patients who have hemophilia or other coagulation disorders
- Heterosexuals who have had sexual contact with someone with AIDS or at risk for AIDS
- Infants who are born to infected mothers

Managing the Cost of HIV and AIDS

The care of an HIV-infected patient, especially when that patient has progressed to AIDS, is one of the most expensive in all of medicine. This is due in part to the fact that the individual drugs are usually very expensive and the patient has to be on multiple drug regimens. The first drug approved to treat HIV was AZT, which cost $10,000 a year when it first came out.

Today, the management of the virus calls for using combination therapy, usually three or even four medications, against the virus. Combination therapy can cost $12,000 a year. Add to that the management of the opportunistic infections and the cost of doctors' visits, tests, and hospitalization and the average cost, as of this writing, of managing an AIDS patient rises to about $20,000 a year or higher for those with advanced diseases.

The current lifetime cost of managing a patient with HIV infection is about $160,000, with the nation now spending about $7 billion a year to take care of those with the virus. This is the direct cost. There are no firm estimates yet on the indirect cost arising from premature death and lost productivity.

About 50 percent of all costs related to HIV medical care is picked up by the government through Medicare (19 percent) and Medicaid (29 percent), with private insurance picking up 32 percent. Twenty percent of HIV-infected patients have no health insurance.

As stated in chapter 1, prevention is always the best way to manage the cost of any disease. It helps to look through numbers:

- The cost of educating high-risk women to avert risky behaviors: $2,000 per infection averted
- The cost of providing free sterile needles: $35,000 per infection averted
- The cost of preventing mother-to-child transmission: $33,000 per infection averted

When you compare these amounts to the $160,000 that it will cost to take care of someone who becomes infected, you realize the significant savings. It has been estimated that the CDC can actually save money from its HIV/AIDS budget by preventing just 1,300 infections a year.

Direct Costs

Direct costs include costs for:

- Physician visits
- Medications
- Institutional care

Physician Visits

As stated previously, the symptoms of early HIV infection can present in a lot of diseases. However, if these symptoms persist (that is, they do not go away after two weeks or more), then the individual should see a doctor, who will test for the presence of HIV. Your doctor will take a history that might involve some very intimate questions about your lifestyle. The answers are important in figuring out if you have been involved in any behaviors that put you at risk for contracting the virus. Your doctor will then do a physical. The diagnosis of HIV is done by checking for the presence of the virus in the blood. There are tests that can be done using oral secretions or urine, but the most effective test is checking the blood for the presence of antibodies to HIV. Antibodies are substances that the body produces to fight germs. There are two specific tests for HIV antibodies: the ELISA and Western blot test. If an ELISA test is positive, then a Western blot test is done to confirm the diagnosis.

At the early stages of infection, the body might not have had the time to produce antibodies. An ELISA or Western blot test at this time might produce a false result. There are other tests that can check the blood for the virus itself.

Once someone has been diagnosed as HIV-positive, the person will visit the doctor as needed, to check for the degree of infection and monitor for opportunistic infections.

Checking for the degree of infections involves monitoring the viral load and the T4 cell count. The higher the viral load, the more virus is in the blood; the lower the T4 cell count (below 200), the more the chances of opportunistic infections. Other tests such as X rays and even scans of the brain and other organs, as well as tests for germs, are done to assess the level of opportunistic infections. These results let the doctor know what treatments to institute.

Individuals with health insurance will have the costs covered through their policies and will have to pay the usual copays or deductibles. Be careful to follow the directions laid out by the plan in regard to which doctors you see. Those in HMO plans should be especially careful about seeing an out-of-plan doctor, since they might have to pay for the visit out of pocket.

If You Do Not Have Insurance

For the 20 percent of HIV-infected individuals without insurance, it is important to keep in mind that care for an AIDS patient can be expensive and intensive. It is also important to see a doctor who has expertise in treating AIDS, and this might mean being seen by a specialist in infectious diseases. A lot of primary care physicians are not comfortable managing AIDS patients. The good news is that the level of advocacy and support for individuals with HIV infection is one of the strongest of any of the chronic diseases. Call your state health office, or any of the resources or advocacy groups listed at the end of this chapter, and inquire about physician services in your area that serve patients with HIV infections. There are many federal, state, and local programs directed specifically to HIV care.

Community and neighborhood clinics usually have federal funding to provide care for the uninsured and underinsured. They can serve as a source of routine care, as well as provide appropriate referral if needed.

Medications

As stated previously, the cost of medications for managing HIV infections is one of the steepest of any disease. The drugs for managing the virus itself are known as anti-retrovirals (ARVs). There are three types of ARVs:

- Nonnucleoside reverse transcriptase inhibitors (NNRTIs)
- Nucleoside analogues reverse transcriptase inhibitors (NRTIs)
- Protease inhibitors (PIs)

Current treatment recommendations call for using a combination of three or more drugs, one of which is a PI. This therapy is known as the Highly Active Anti-Retroviral Therapy (HAART). Patients usually take as many as 30 pills a day, at different times, with or without food. One of the ways drug companies are trying to reduce this burden is to make drugs that already combine some of the medicines.

Patients also have to worry about developing resistance to the drug; that is, the drug might stop being effective. They then have to try a new combination. Unfortunately, sometimes they can run out of combinations.

The following table shows the different ARVs. As of this writing, their costs vary considerably, from about $250 to well above $850 for a month's supply for one drug. And these drugs have to be taken in combination. HIV/AIDs is, therefore, one of the most expensive conditions to manage.

Class	Brand Names	Cost of a Month's Starting Dose	Manufacturer*
Nonnucleoside reverse transcriptase inhibitors (NNRTIs)	Rescriptor	$285	Agouron
	Sustiva	$385	DuPont
	Viramune	$313	Roxane
Nucleoside analogues reverse transcriptase inhibitors (NRTIs)	Epivir	$267	GlaxoSmithKline
	Hivid	$242	Roche
	Retrovir (AZT)	$322	GlaxoSmithKline
	Videx	$298	Bristol-Myers Squibb
	Zerit	$327	Bristol-Myers Squibb
	Ziagen	$354	GlaxoSmithKline
Protease inhibitors (PIs)	Agenerase	$660	GlaxoSmithKline
	Crixivan	$526	GlaxoSmithKline
	Invirase	$635	Roche
	Norvir	$702	Abbott
	Viracept	$633	Agouron
Combination	Combivir	$602	GlaxoSmithKline
	Kaletra	$852	Abbott
	Trizivir	$1,044	GlaxoSmithKline

*See appendix B for the phone numbers of the manufacturers.

Drug prices can vary by neighborhood, although the difference in cost among drugs will be about the same. While you should be aware of the differences in prices and discuss them with your doctor, remember that these drugs are very tricky to administer and manage and hence you might not have a lot of leeway to practice brand substitution. This is especially true if you start developing resistance to the drugs.

Programs to Assist with the Cost of HIV Medications

Several agencies and programs can assist with the cost of HIV medications. They include Medicaid, Medicare, the Ryan White National AIDS Drug Assistance Program (ADAP), and drug company patient assistance programs.

Medicaid. Medicaid is the largest payer of prescriptions for those with HIV. It is estimated that 55 percent of those with HIV are enrolled in Medicaid. (See chapter 1 for information on Medicaid eligibility.) Also check with your state's health office to determine if you are eligible for Medicaid, either because of your income level or because you are disabled. HIV is a disease that results in disability. Disability, for purposes of insurance, is when an individual cannot engage in a "substantial gainful activity by reason of a medically determined physical or mental impairment expected to result in death, or has lasted or can be expected to last for a continuous period for at least 12 months." Because of an HIV infection, you might stop working and the drop of your income would make you qualify for Medicaid. A lot of people with AIDS qualify for Medicaid because of their disability rather than their income. Many low-income individuals who do not yet meet the income qualification might have to wait some time before Medicaid kicks in. During this interval, they might forgo drug therapy because of the cost and yet the guidelines for their treatment might require them to be on medications. The Ticket to Work and Work Incentives Improvement Act (TWWIIA) or Welfare Reform Act of 1999 allow low-income individuals with disabilities to work while allowing them to keep their Medicaid coverage. This might help an AIDS patient get Medicaid even if he or she is still working.

Medicare. In general, Medicare does not cover prescription drugs. If you have a Medicare HMO, you might have prescription drug coverage as part of your package. Most Medicare recipients with HIV also qualify for Medicaid and so get their prescription drugs through Medicaid.

The Ryan White National AIDS Drug Assistance Program. The Ryan White Comprehensive AIDS Resources Emergency (CARE) Act was passed in 1990 and reauthorized in 1996 and again in 2000, to provide assistance to states, cities, and private organizations helping with the fight against HIV infection. Title II of the Act supports the ADAP, which is an assistance of last resort for those who are uninsured or underinsured and do not qualify for Medicaid. It is run through the states and each state has a lot of leeway in designing its own program. This has resulted in different criteria for eligibility in different states, and in a difference in the number and type of drugs that are covered. For example, the maximum income level for qualification in Massachusetts in 2001 was $32,200 a year, while in New York it was $44,000. The number of drugs covered also varies from 20 to as high as 100. Since the program is administered through the state's Medicaid office, contact your state health office for eligibility criteria and coverage.

Drug Company Patient Assistance Programs. Drug companies are aware of the fact that many of the drugs to fight HIV and the opportunistic infections are expensive. They also recognize that because most individuals with AIDS are taking numerous medications, the cost of medicines can present a financial burden. Nearly all the companies that make HIV and related medicines have programs to assist individuals with the cost of medications. Appendix B lists the phone numbers of the various manufacturers.

Clinical Trials and Compassionate Use

Clinical trials for HIV medications are another way to get free drugs. Be aware, however, that in certain drug trials, known as double-blind trials, the patient and the physician do not know if the patient is taking an active medication or just a dummy pill. Be aware also of the risks involved and be sure to understand fully all aspects of the trial. Then and only then should you give your informed consent to participate in the trial. To find out about clinical trials, log onto the National Institute of Health's web site at http://clinicaltrials.gov or call (301) 496-4000.

Another way to get free drugs is through the compassionate use program. In this program, individuals are given free medications even though the drug is still undergoing testing. This is not a trial. In this case, the drug has been shown to work and the individuals are being given the active medication while the government is still reviewing the results and preparing to approve it officially. Ask your doctor about this program.

Discount Pharmacy Programs

All the discount pharmacy programs described in chapter 5 can be used to realize savings on HIV and other medications. Buyer's Clubs also have sprung up in various cities to help individuals with HIV learn more about different programs that can assist them with medication costs. These buyer's clubs also educate individuals on the importation of drugs for personal use. The most active clubs are in New York, San Francisco, Boston, and Phoenix. To find out about one in your area, call the Gay Men's Health Crisis at (800) 243-7692.

Private Insurance

Most private insurance comes through employers. Individuals with HMO or indemnity coverage get their medications through the plan and pay a copay or deductible as the case may be. The issue with individuals who are HIV-positive comes when someone has to change jobs and would thus need to get new health insurance. The fear is that the preexisting condition would prevent getting coverage. People in this category are protected from this by both the HIPAA law, which governs insurance for those with preexisting conditions, and COBRA, which protects people from losing their insurance because they changed jobs. Chapter 8 describes these laws in detail. The Ryan White CARE Act can assist individuals with payment of premiums under COBRA.

Veteran Affairs (VA) and Department of Defense (DOD)

The Veteran Affairs (VA) is one of the largest providers of care for individuals with HIV and AIDS. It cares for about 50,000 individuals with the virus. The Department of Defense (DOD) also provides care to a number of personnel who are still on active duty. Contact the proper agency if you served in the military.

Institutional Care

AIDS patients end up in the hospital because of one or more opportunistic infections. Hospital stays involve aggressive therapy to eradicate the body of the invading organism. Stays in the hospital for AIDS patients do not usually result in procedures, so much of the cost arises from physician visits and special services that might be provided to accommodate needs, like special nutrition.

Those with insurance, should review their policy to know what is and what is not covered under the plan. Those without insurance should review chapter 7 to explore ways to get help with the cost of hospitalization.

Indirect Costs

Indirect costs of any disease arise from lost productivity from missed workdays and premature death. Individuals with HIV and AIDS have protections under the Americans with Disabilities Act (ADA), so an employer cannot discriminate against someone with the virus. An individual with HIV should enjoy all the benefits that all other employees enjoy. The ADA also requires the employer to make reasonable accommodations to allow the person to perform the essential functions of the job. Federal government employees get the same rights through the Rehabilitation Act.

The Family Leave Act allows HIV and AIDS patients to take up to 12 weeks of unpaid leave to take care of themselves, without fear of losing their jobs.

Intangible Cost

One of the biggest costs in dealing with HIV and AIDS is that of relationships. HIV infection is one of the most stigmatized diseases and leaves a lot of infected individuals feeling ashamed and rejected. Because of misconceptions that one can catch the virus by being near someone with HIV, many individuals refuse to go near anyone with the virus. While an individual with HIV has to make certain changes, like making sure there is protection if there is to be intimate contact with another person, he or she should be able to live as normal a life as those without the virus.

As with any other chronic disease and even more so with HIV infection, educating those with the disease as well as those around them is essential to establishing a relationship free of worries or prejudices.

Complementary and Alternative Medicine

A number of products have been used to complement, and in some cases used in place of (alternative), conventional therapy. The buyer's clubs have been very instrumental in educating individuals about these therapies and how to obtain them. Some of the most widely used products are:

DHEA. Dehydro-3-epiandrosterone, known widely as DHEA, is a naturally occurring steroid that is diminished in individuals with HIV. These decreased levels could be responsible for the wasting that is often observed in AIDS patients. DHEA is widely used by HIV-positive persons and even by HIV-negative individuals to increase body mass. It is also thought to have anti-aging, anti-obesity, and anti-cancer properties.

Ketotifen. This antihistamine is thought to help with wasting. It is also believed to stimulate appetite and to have anti-inflammatory properties.

Marijuana. This is used as an appetite stimulant and there are studies under way to see if it has beneficial effects on the immune system. Because marijuana is an illicit drug, there are many legal hurdles to overcome for it to have any level of widespread use.

Vitamins and supplements. The antioxidant vitamins A, C, E, as well as beta-carotene, zinc, selenium, glutathione, and coenzyme Q-10, are widely used to help boost the body's immune system.

NAC. N-acetylcysteine is one of a number of products thought to inhibit a substance called tumor necrosis factor (TNF). TNF has been shown to increase the activity of HIV and the belief is that if TNF is suppressed, the HIV will be less active.

Chinese Medicine. Acupuncture and Chinese herbs are being used in some AIDS patients. Two widely used Chinese medicines are Clear Heat and Enhance. Each one is made up of several different herbs.

Note: Not all the therapies described here have been adequately investigated. When any complementary or alternative therapy is being used or considered, inform your physician about it to avoid the risk of drug interactions with a prescription medication.

Resources

For information about
FDA-approved HIV trials
(800) 874-2572
www.actis.org

For FDA-approved treatments
(800) 448-0440
www.hivatis.org

For prevention materials
National Prevention Information
Network
(800) 458-5231
www.cdcnpin.org

Centers for Disease Control
National AIDS Hotline: (800)
342-2437
For HIV/AIDS Information (800)
311-3435
www.cdc.org

National Minority AIDS Council
(202) 483-6622
www.nmac.org

For confidential AIDS treatment
issues
Project Inform: (800) 822-7422
www.projinf.org

National Association of People
with AIDS
(202) 898-0414
www.napwa.org

American Foundation for AIDS
Research (AMFAR)
(800) 392-6327
www.amfar.org

Gay Men's Health Crisis
(800) 243-7692
www.gmhc.org

ACT UP
Local chapters include:
Philadelphia
(215) 731-1844
www.critpath.org/actup

New York
(212) 966-4873
www.actupny.org

San Francisco
(415) 864-6686
www.actupsf.org

Washington, D.C.
(202) 547-9404
www.actupdc.org

CHAPTER 17

Osteoporosis

A t present, more than 28 million North Americans have gone over the so-called fracture threshold—that is, their bone densities have been reduced to the point where they can easily break. Of these, about 10 million already have osteoporosis, a condition that causes severe loss of bone mass, making the bones brittle. It affects women more than men, and of the 10 million cited, 8 million are women.

What makes osteoporosis a costly disease is the fact that it results in fractures of bones, mostly the hip, and that is very costly to manage. About 25 percent of hip fracture patients 50 years and older die a year after their fractures. One out of every two women and one out of every eight men over 50 will have an osteoporosis-related fracture in his or her lifetime, according to the National Osteoporosis Foundation.

What Is Osteoporosis?

Bone is constantly being added and broken down at the same time. There are cells that add on to bone and cells that break down bone. These cells are affected by many chemicals in our bodies, especially the sex hormones estrogen and testosterone. As we grow, the thickness or density of our bones increases. This continues until our 30s, at which time we have the greatest bone density. The density level stays that way for about 10 years and then slowly starts to decline, because as we get older and the chemicals in our bodies that lead to bone loss change (e.g., the level of estrogen declines in menopause), the rate at which bone is broken down becomes greater than the rate at which bone is made. As this occurs, the bone density is gradually reduced. Bone loss continues and puts us at a risk for bones breaking. The rate of decline is greater in women than in men at first. However, by age 70 both men and women lose bone at the same rate. Men not only catch up to women but by age 75 men are three times more likely to die from a hip fracture than are women.

Symptoms

Osteoporosis is a "silent" disease. For most people, the first indication that they have osteoporosis is when a major fracture occurs. In some individuals, minor fractures, especially of the spine, will occur, causing them to feel a sharp pain that feels worse if weight is added, and might decrease after about a week. As more and more fractures occur in the spine, the pain becomes chronic, dull, and aching, especially in the lower back.

Another sign of osteoporosis is that of losing height. As bone loss in the spine progresses, the spine becomes deformed and the patient starts developing a stooped posture, a condition known clinically as kyphosis.

Prevention

While osteoporosis can be severely damaging and painful, the good news is that it is one of those chronic diseases that we know a lot about preventing. With proper precautions and steps taken to prevent bone loss, osteoporosis can not only be delayed but also completely prevented. The five major ways to prevent osteoporosis are:

- Diet
- Exercise
- Avoiding lifestyle choices that can cause bone lose
- Avoiding medications that can cause bone loss
- Routine physical examinations

Diet

Calcium is needed to make bones. The body actually needs calcium for a lot more activities than just making bones; it needs calcium for skeletal muscles to contract, for the heart to beat, and for nerves to conduct. If you can't absorb the calcium you take in with your food, the body will steal calcium from your bones. While everyone needs calcium to keep the bones strong, it is needed even more through those years when the rate of bone loss starts to exceed the rate of bone formation. The National Academy of Science (NAS) has recommended that individuals from age 31 to 50 get 1,000 mg of calcium a day. Individuals over age 50 should take in 1,200 mg of calcium a day. You get the calcium you need through calcium supplements or from the foods you eat.

To get the calcium you need from foods, include in your meals more of the following:

- Low-fat dairy foods such as cheese, yogurt, and low-fat milk
- Canned fish with bones you can eat, such as salmon and sardines
- Dark-green leafy vegetables, such as kale, collards, and broccoli
- Calcium-fortified orange juice
- Breads made with calcium-fortified flour

To get 1,200 mg of calcium you should eat three to four servings each day of dairy foods. A serving is a cup of milk or yogurt, 11/2 ounces of cheese, or 2 cups of cottage cheese.

If you need to take supplements, as most people should, it is advised that you do not take more than 500 mg at once in the beginning. This gives your body a chance to get used to it. Calcium in the form of calcium carbonate should be taken with food and calcium citrate can be taken any time. Choose brand-name supplements since these are purified and more easily absorbed. As with all supplement consumption, tell your doctor about your use of calcium, since it can interact with some medications.

Vitamin D is another element that should be taken to help prevent osteoporosis. The body needs vitamin D to absorb calcium. The recommended amount of vitamin D is 400 IU (international units) per day for people age 51 to 70 and 600 IU for people over age 70. Individuals should not take more than 2,000 IU of vitamin D a day since this might lead to liver damage.

You can get vitamin D from three sources:

- Being in the sun for about 20 minutes a day
- Foods such as eggs, fatty fish, liver, milk, and cereal fortified with vitamins
- Calcium supplements that include vitamin D

Exercise

Another proven way to prevent osteoporosis is to exercise. The younger that one starts an exercise program, the longer one can maintain bone density. However, it is never too late to begin. The recommended regimen for an exercise program to strengthen bones is to do weight-bearing exercise three to four times a week. The following exercises are weight-bearing exercises:

- Dancing
- Hiking
- Jogging
- Tennis
- Racquetball
- Stair climbing
- Walking

Remember to follow the guidelines suggested in chapter 2 when exercising. As a reminder, be sure to start with a low-intensity program before proceeding to a more vigorous activity. Also, be sure to discuss your exercise program with your doctor, especially if you are frail, have not exercised in a long time, or have a medical condition that might affect your exercise program.

Avoiding Lifestyle Choices That Can Cause Bone Loss

Certain activities can cause bone loss. Prolonged involvement in these lifestyles puts you at risk for osteoporosis and bone fractures. Avoid these activities:

- Smoking, which causes your body to make less estrogen
- Excess alcohol, which can damage your bones

Avoiding Medications That Can Cause Bone Loss

Some medications can cause loss of bone density. They include:

- Glucocorticoids (steroids taken to treat such conditions as arthritis and asthma)
- Sleeping pills
- Antiseizure drugs

- Hormones for endometriosis
- Some cancer drugs

If you are taking any of these medications, do not stop taking them. You should, however, discuss with your doctor about their bone loss effect and see if there are substitutes or things that can be done to counteract their bone-decreasing effect.

Routine Physical Examinations

As stated previously, osteoporosis is truly a silent disease. The only way to tell if you have osteoporosis, or are losing bone at a rate that puts you at risk for osteoporosis, is to get a bone mass measurement. The hope is to catch bone loss early enough to take precautionary measures and avoid falls and bone fractures. It is a lot more expensive to deal with bone fractures than to monitor bone loss.

High-Risk Factors

Certain risk factors put one in a position to be more likely to develop osteoporosis. According to the National Osteoporosis Foundation, the following are risk factors:

- Being female
- Being thin or having a small frame
- Advanced age
- A family history of osteoporosis
- Postmenopause, including early or surgically induced menopause
- Abnormal absence of menstrual period
- Anorexia nervosa or bulimia
- A diet low in calcium
- Use of medications that can cause bone loss
- Low testosterone in men
- Inactive lifestyle
- Cigarette smoking
- Excessive use of alcohol
- Being white or Asian

If you have any of these risk factors, you should discuss with your doctor your risk of having osteoporosis. You should set a schedule for regular bone mass testing, and more important, start taking the steps discussed previously to reduce the rate of bone loss.

Managing the Cost

The total cost of managing osteoporosis has not yet been determined. The nursing home care and hospitalization costs to deal with osteoporosis and the resulting fractures were estimated to be almost $24 billion in 1995. More than 1.5 million fractures occur each year because of osteoporosis. These fractures are broken down as follows:

- 300,000 hip fractures
- 700,000 fractures of the spine
- 250,000 wrist fractures
- 300,000 fractures from other sites

It is thought that the cost of managing osteoporosis is much higher because many more resources are spent to deal with direct costs like medical services and products as well as other costs incurred at home to accommodate a patient who has suffered fractures and might need a modified lifestyle. Dietary supplements and other lifestyle modifications designed to prevent osteoporosis also add to the cost of the disease.

Direct Costs

The direct costs of osteoporosis come mostly from:
- Physician visits and tests
- Medication
- Institutional care

Physician Visits and Tests

Your doctor can perform several tests to determine what is happening to the rate of bone loss in your body. He or she might check your blood and urine for calcium activity. The single most important test, however, is a bone mineral density (BMD) test. The BMD test measures your bone mass and compares the results to two normal readings, an aged-matched reading where the result is compared to people of your age, sex, and size, and a "young normal" match where your result is compared to those of young healthy adults of the same sex. The results are reported as a deviation from the standard (standard deviation or SD).

A result of –1SD to –2.5SD means you have some bone loss and are at risk to develop osteoporosis. A result of –2.5SD or greater means you have osteoporosis.

Different types of scans measure bone density at different parts of the body. The DEXA (dual energy X-ray absorptiometry) is a whole-body scan and can generate results for the hip and or spine bones. It is the standard measurement for bone density. Other scans are used to measure bone density in the wrist, heel, shinbone, or finger. These tests are painless, take very little time, and are very safe.

The tests cost between $75 and $150. If you have insurance, your doctor visits and tests will be covered. If you have already been diagnosed with osteoporosis, then your tests and doctor visits are considered part of treating a disease for which you have coverage. The issue is when you visit a doctor and get tests for prevention purposes as opposed to treatment purposes. Fortunately, most insurance companies recognize the importance of prevention and will pay for these tests and visits. In fact, as of July 1998, Medicare started paying for preventive BMD tests. Medicare allows bone testing every two years, or more frequently if a doctor determines that it is necessary.

If You Do Not Have Insurance

If you do not have insurance, call around for less expensive tests. The important thing to remember is that these tests are all useful and can detect bone loss but are more effective if you have them done consistently. You need to keep a history so that your bone loss progression can be followed. These tests also help to determine the effectiveness of preventive measures, as well as treatments.

Medications

The following classes of drugs have been approved for the treatment for osteoporosis. The prices of these drugs differ considerably.

Class	Brand Names	Cost of a Month's Starting Dose	Manufacturer*
Bisphosphonates	Actonel	$443	Procter & Gamble
	Fosamax	$69	Merck

(continued)

(continued)

Class	Brand Names	Cost of a Month's Starting Dose	Manufacturer*
Calcitonin	Miacalcin	$69	Novartis
Estrogen	Estrace	$9	Warner Chilcott
	Estraderm	$25	Novartis
	Estratab	$17	Solvay
	Femhrt	$26	Pfizer
	Ogen	$26	Pharmacia
	Ortho-Prefest	$29	Ortho-McNeil
	Premarin	$19	Wyeth
	Premphase	$35	Wyeth
	Prempro	$38	Wyeth
	Vivelle	$37	Novartis
Selective Estrogen Receptor Modulator (SERM)	Evista	$62	Lilly

*See appendix B for the phone number of the manufacturer.

Strategies to manage the cost of osteoporosis medications include the following:

Brand-Name Substitution

As you can see from the previous chart, there are different classes of drugs used to treat osteoporosis. They work in different ways:

- Bisphosphonates slow down the rate at which bone is broken down and can also increase bone density.
- Calcitonin is a naturally occurring hormone that increases bone mass.
- Estrogen helps to slow down the rate of bone loss. Estrogen Replacement Therapy (ERT) is used to replace the estrogen that is lost as a result of menopause.
- Selective Estrogen Receptor Modulators work by making the existing estrogen in the body more effective.

Within each class, there are usually different drugs. All of these drugs have been shown to be effective in treating osteoporosis. The prices can vary considerably between the classes and within the class. If your doctor determines that one class might be better for you, it might be wise to start with the least expensive one, unless there is a reason not to.

Generic Substitution

At the present time, a few generic drugs are available to combat osteoporosis. While there are some estrogen generics available, estrogens are very tricky to administer, so physicians are careful about using generics.

Pill Cutting

Some of the medications for osteoporosis cannot be cut. Most estrogens, for example, come as patches that should not be tampered with. Others come as combinations and pill cutting might tamper with the combination. There are, however, certain drugs for osteoporosis that are available as tablets. The prices are usually the same for the different strengths so if you are at a lower dose, ask your doctor to prescribe the higher dose and then split it. You should ask for assistance from your pharmacist to make sure you are doing it correctly.

Drug Company Assistance Programs

Appendix B provides the phone numbers of the various manufacturers. If a manufacturer is not listed, then as of this writing that manufacturer does not provide a patient assistance program. If you have been prescribed any of these products and you cannot afford them, call the manufacturer and explain your situation. If you need help in navigating the process, call one of the companies listed in chapter 5 for assistance.

Other Strategies to Reduce Medication Costs

Revisit chapters 4 and 5 for other strategies like samples, mail order, discount programs, and state government programs. Use as many as you can. The more programs you use the more savings you will achieve.

Institutional Care

The most serious and significant complications to arise from osteoporosis are the fractures that result when the weakened bones break. When a fracture occurs, especially in weight-bearing bones like the spine and the hip, the patient ends up in a hospital for either repairs or replacement. Hip-replacement surgeries are now one of the most common surgeries in hospitals and are second only to stroke as the most common reason for a patient being discharged to another institution, in this case, either to a rehabilitation facility or to a nursing home. The strategies for dealing with institutional care are described in chapter 7.

Since about one-fourth of all patients age 50 and older who have had a hip fracture die in the year following the fracture, the end-of-life issues as discussed in chapter 8 should be considered. This involves various legal and financial planning to reduce the impact of a loved one passing away.

Indirect Costs

The indirect costs of osteoporosis are not so much related to economics of lost production but rather to the emotional burdens of seeing a loved one reduced to a helpless state if he or she ends up in a nursing home or rehabilitation facility. There are caregiver issues related to osteoporosis as is seen in the care of the Alzheimer's patient. Caregiver support groups are therefore essential if your loved one has developed complications from osteoporosis.

Resources

National Institute on Aging
   (NIA)
(800) 222-2225
www.nih.gov/nia

National Osteoporosis
   Foundation
(202) 223-2226
www.nof.org

Directory of State Health and Insurance Agencies

States with Prescription Assistance Programs

All programs, eligibility qualifications, and program descriptions are as of 2002. Log on to www.ncol-org/programs/health for updates on these programs.

ALASKA
The Chronic and Acute Medical Assistance
(CAMA) program

Eligibility	• Alaska resident.
	• Does not qualify for Medicaid.
	• Income requirements must be met. Call for specifics.
	• Has no other resources to pay medical bills.
	• Has less than $500 in personal resources not counting home, income-producing property, or car.
How the Program Works	• First apply to CAMA before seeking care unless in an emergency.
	• Produce a doctor's statement that you need care.
	• Once approved, you receive a coupon to present at the pharmacy when filling the prescription.
Cost to Join	None.
Copay	None.
Drugs Covered	Drugs for chemotherapy, diabetes, seizure disorders, mental illness, or hypertension.
Contact Number	(888) 804-6330

Alaska Division of Insurance   (907) 269-7900

CALIFORNIA
Prescription Assistance for Medicare Patients

Eligibility	• California resident.
	• Enrolled in Medicare.
How the Program Works	• Present the Medicare card at any pharmacy participating in the MediCal Program.
	• Receive the drug at MediCal Rates.
Cost to Join	None.
Copay	15-cent processing fee per prescription.
Drugs Covered	All drugs on the MediCal Formulary.
Contact Number	(916) 445-5014

California Department of Insurance   (213) 897-8921

CONNECTICUT
Connecticut Pharmaceutical Assistance Contract to the Elderly (ConnPACE)

Eligibility	• Age 65 and older, or disabled and age 18 or older.
	• Connecticut resident for at least 6 months.
	• Income requirements must be met. Call for specifics.
	• No other insurance covering drugs or reached limit on other drug plan.
How the Program Works	• Call for an application and apply.
	• Receive card after approval.
	• Present the card at the pharmacy when filling a prescription.
	• Pay a copay.
Cost to Join	Annual fee of $25.
Copay	$12 per prescription.
Drugs Covered	Most drugs except antihistamines, contraceptives, and experimental drugs.
Contact Number	(800) 842-1508

Connecticut Department of Insurance   (800) 203-3447

DELAWARE
Delaware Prescription Assistance Program

Eligibility	• Age 65 and older.
	• Income requirements must be met. Call for specifics.
	• Individuals under age 65 but eligible for Social Security Disability (SSDI).
	• Elderly and disabled with higher incomes but drug costs are over 40% of yearly income.
How the Program Works	• Apply and get a card.
	• Present the card at any participating pharmacy.

- Receive the drug at Medicaid cost.
- Program pays up to $2,500 per person per year.

Cost to Join	None.
Copay	$5 or 25% of cost, whichever is greater.
Drugs Covered	Drugs from all manufacturers that have agreed to the state's rebate program.
Contact Number	(800) 996-9969, ext. 17

The Nemours Foundation (private)

Eligibility	• Age 65 and older. • Income requirements must be met. Call for specifics.
How the Program Works	• Senior or representative with patient's card takes the prescription to the Nemours clinic (1801 Rockland Road, Wilmington, DE 19803) or to one of their satellite clinics. • Pay only 20% of drug's cost.
Cost to Join	None.
Copay	20% of drug's cost.
Drugs Covered	Most drugs.
Contact Number	(800) 292-9538

Delaware Department of Insurance   (800) 282-8611

FLORIDA
Pharmaceutical Expense Assistance for Low-Income Elderly

Eligibility	• Florida resident. • Age 65 and older. • Eligible for Medicare. • Not enrolled in a Medicare HMO with pharmacy benefits. • Income requirements must be met. Call for specifics. • Reached limit on insurance plan. • Insurance does not cover a particular drug.
How the Program Works	• Present Medicare card and proof of Florida residency at any pharmacy that accepts Medicaid. • Get the drug at discounted prices subject to the Senior Prescription Affordability Act.
Cost to Join	None.
Copay	None.
Drugs Covered	All prescriptions.
Contact Number	(888) 419-3456

Florida Department of Insurance   (800) 342-2762

ILLINOIS
Circuit Breaker and Pharmaceutical Assistance Program

Eligibility	• Age 65 years and older, or disabled and age 16 or older.
	• Income requirements must be met. Call for specifics.
How the Program Works	• Apply and get a card.
	• Present the card to the pharmacy when picking up the prescription.
	• Pay the wholesale price minus 20%.
	• Program pays up to $2,000 for the year, after which the patient pays 20% of the cost of the prescription.
Cost to Join	$5 or $25, based on income.
Copay	• No copay if your cost to join is $5.
	• $3 if your cost to join is $25.
Drugs Covered	Drugs for arthritis, Alzheimer's disease, cancer, diabetes, glaucoma, heart diseases, Parkinson's, and smoking-related illnesses.
Contact Number	(800) 356-6302

Illinois Department of Insurance   (312) 814-2427

INDIANA
HoosierRx Program

Eligibility	• Indiana resident.
	• Age 65 and older.
	• No insurance coverage for prescription drugs.
	• Income requirements must be met. Call for specifics.
How the Program Works	• Fill in and send application.
	• If eligible, the state mails back refund certificates.
	• Mail back the refund certificates and a printout of the prescription receipt from the pharmacy.
	• Receive a refund check in about 45 days.
	• Refund check is 50% of cost up to $1,000 or $500 per year depending on income.
Cost to Join	None.
Copay	None.
Drugs Covered	All FDA-approved prescriptions.
Contact Number	(866) 267-4679

Indiana Department of Insurance   (317) 232-2385

MAINE
Elderly Low-Cost Drug Program

Eligibility	• Age 62 and older, or disabled and age 19 or older.
	• Monthly income of less than $1,279 per single or $1,705 per couple.
	• If medication is over 40% of household income then income limit is 25% higher than above.
How the Program Works	• Apply and get a card.
	• Present the card when filling a prescription.
	• Pay 20% of the medication's price or $2, whichever is greater, for all generics.
	• After spending $1,000 for the year, you pay 20% or $2, whichever is greater, for all prescriptions.
Cost to Join	None
Copay	$2 if greater than 20% of the drug's cost.
Drugs Covered	Prescriptions for nearly all major chronic illnesses.
Contact Number	(888) 600-2466

Maine Bureau of Insurance   (800) 300-5000

MARYLAND
Maryland Pharmacy Assistance Program (MPAP)

Eligibility	• Maryland resident.
	• All; no age limit.
	• Income less than $9,650 and assets of less than $3,750 for a single person or income less than $10,050 and assets less than $4,500 for household.
How the Program Works	• Apply and get a card.
	• Present the card at the pharmacy with a copay.
Cost to Join	None.
Copay	$5.
Drugs Covered	Chronic maintenance drugs and anti-infectives.
Contact Number	(800) 492-1974

Maryland Insurance Administration   (800) 492-6116

MASSACHUSETTS
Senior Pharmacy Program

Eligibility	• Age 65 and older.
	• Income requirements must be met. Call for specifics.
	• Not enrolled in MassHealth or CommonHealth.
How the Program Works	• Join and receive a card.
	• Annual enrollment fee of $15.

Massachusetts (continued)

* At the pharmacy pay only a copay.
* Benefit capped at $1,250 per year.

Cost to Join   None.

Copay   • $3 for generic.
                        • $10 for brand name.

Drugs Covered   All prescription drugs except those excluded from
                        MassHealth.

Contact Number   (800) 243-4636

Massachusetts Division of Insurance   (617) 521-7777

MICHIGAN
Michigan Emergency Pharmaceutical Program for Seniors (MEPPS)

Eligibility   • Age 65 years and older.
                        • Income requirements must be met. Call for specifics.
                        • Cost of drugs represents 10% or more of single's
                          income or 8% of couple's income.

How the Program Works Once enrolled, at the pharmacy pay the wholesale
                        price less 12%.

Cost to Join   None.

Copay   None. $0.25 per prescription (voluntary).

Drugs Covered   All drugs on state's formulary.

Contact Number   (517) 373-8230

Michigan Insurance Bureau   (877) 999-6442

MINNESOTA
Senior Drug Program

Eligibility   • Age 65 years and older.
                        • Minnesota resident for 6 months.
                        • Income requirements must be met. Call for specifics.
                        • No prescription coverage within four months of
                          applying.
                        • Not enrolled in MinnesotaCare.
                        • Not living in a nursing home.

How the Program Works • Once enrolled, at the pharmacy pay wholesale price
                          less 9%.
                        • Program is used after $35 monthly deductible.

Cost to Join   None.

Copay $3.

Drugs Covered   Drugs on state's formulary, plus vitamins.

Contact Number   (800) 333-2433

Minnesota Insurance Division   (800) 657-3602

NEVADA
SeniorRx

Eligibility	• Nevada resident for at least 1 year.
	• Age 62 and older.
	• Not eligible for Medicaid.
	• Income requirements must be met. Call for specifics.
How the Program Works	• Obtain an application and chose one of two plans, basic or enhanced plan.
	• The state subsidizes the drug insurance premium based on income, ranging from $24.58 to $40 per month.
	• The premium covers the drug benefit for up to $5,000 per year.
Cost to Join	• Premiums are based on income through Fidelity Security Life Insurance/Professional Risk and Asset Management Insurance Services (PRAM).
Copay	$10 per prescription.
Drugs Covered	All prescription drugs.
Contact Number	(800) 262-7726

Nevada Insurance Division   (775) 687-4270

NEW HAMPSHIRE
New Hampshire Senior Prescription Drug Discount Program

Eligibility	• New Hampshire resident.
	• Age 65 or older.
	• No income eligibility.
How the Program Works	• Apply and receive a card.
	• Take the prescription to a participating pharmacy.
	• Receive medication on a discount of up to 15% for brand drugs and 40% for generics.
Cost to Join	None.
Copay	None.
Drugs Covered	All prescription drugs.
Contact Number	(603) 271-4688

New Hampshire Insurance Department   (800) 852-3416

NEW JERSEY
Pharmaceutical Assistance to the Aged and Disabled (PAAD)

Eligibility	• New Jersey resident for at least 30 days.
	• Age 65 and older or disabled and age 18 or older.
	• Income requirements must be met. Call for specifics.

New Jersey (continued)

How the Program Works	• Get an application through various senior centers or local pharmacies, or call for an application.
	• Once enrolled, present the card at any participating pharmacy.
	• Obtain medication with only a copay.
Cost to Join	None.
Copay	$5 per prescription.
Drugs Covered	All prescription drugs.
Contact Number	(800) 792-9745

New Jersey Department of Banking and Insurance   (800) 838-0935

NEW YORK
Elderly Pharmaceutical Insurance Coverage (EPIC) Fee Plan

Eligibility	• Age 65 years and older.
	• Income requirements must be met. Call for specifics.
How the Program Works	• Enroll and choose the fee plan.
	• Present the card at the pharmacy.
	• Pay a copay.
	• Annual fees range from $8 to $230 for a single person, or $8 to $300 for married couples, based on income.
Cost to Join	Pay fees stated above.
Copay	Between $3 and $20 per prescription based on cost of prescription.
Drugs Covered	All drugs from the manufacturers participating in program.
Contact Number	(800) 332-3724

EPIC Deductible Plan

Eligibility	• Age 65 and older.
	• Income requirements must be met. Call for specifics.
How the Program Works	• Enroll and choose the deductible plan.
	• Present the card at the pharmacy and pay a copay for the rest of the year after meeting the yearly deductible.
	• Deductibles range from $530 to $ 1,230 for a single person, or $650 to $1,715 for married couples, based on income.
Cost to Join	None.
Copay	Between $3 and $23, depending on the cost of the drug.
Drugs Covered	All drugs from the manufacturers participating in the program.

Contact Number   (800) 332-3742

New York Insurance Department   (800) 342-3736

PENNSYLVANIA
Pharmaceutical Assistance for the Elderly (PACE)
Eligibility	• Pennsylvania resident for at least 90 days.
	• Age 65 and older.
	• Income requirements must be met. Call for specifics.
How the Program Works	• Enroll.
	• Present the card at the pharmacy.
	• Pay a copay.
Cost to Join	None.
Copay	$6 per prescription.
Drugs Covered	Most prescription drugs.
Contact Number	(800) 225-7223

PACE Needs Enhancement Tier (PACENET)
Eligibility	• Age 65 and older.
	• Yearly income less than $16,000 for a single person or $19,200 for a married couple.
How the Program Works	• Enroll.
	• Satisfy an annual deductible of $500.
	• Present the card at the pharmacy and pay a copay.
Cost to Join	None.
Copay	$8 for generics, $15 for brand names per prescription.
Drugs Covered	Most prescriptions.
Contact Number	(800) 225-7223

Pennsylvania Insurance Department   (877) 881-6388

RHODE ISLAND
Rhode Island Pharmaceutical Assistance for the Elderly (RIPAE)
Eligibility	• Age 65 and older.
	• Income requirements must be met. Call for specifics.
How the Program Works	• Enroll.
	• Reach the limit on insurance coverage, or no insurance.
	• Present the card at pharmacy.
	• Buy the drug at a discount.
Cost to Join	None.
Copay	Between 40% and 85% of retail cost.

Rhode Island (continued)

Drugs Covered	Medication for high blood pressure, heart disease, high cholesterol, asthma, chronic respiratory disease, diabetes, cancer, Parkinson's disease, glaucoma, Alzheimer's disease.
Contact Number	(401) 222-2858

Rhode Island Insurance Division   (401) 222-2223

SOUTH CAROLINA
SilverRxCard

Eligibility	• South Carolina resident for 6 months. • Age 65 and older. • Not on Medicaid. • Income requirements must be met. Call for specifics.
How the Program Works	• Apply during the open enrollment period or if you qualify, in the course of the year. • After the yearly deductible is met, use the card at a participating pharmacy. • Pay copay for prescription.
Cost to Join	None.
Copay	$10 for generics, $21 for brand name drugs per 30-day period.
Drugs Covered	All FDA-approved prescriptions.
Contact Number	(877) 239-5277

South Carolina Department of Insurance   (803) 737-6231

VERMONT
Vermont Health Access Plan (VHAP)—Pharmacy

Eligibility	• Age 65 and older. • Income requirements must be met. Call for specifics. • Disabled and receiving benefits through Social Security or Medicare.
How the Program Works	• Submit an application. • Pay a premium of no more than $25 per 6 months. • Present the card at the pharmacy and pay a copay.
Cost to Join	None.
Copay	$1 for prescriptions costing less than $29.99 and $2 for prescriptions costing more than $30.
Drugs Covered	All prescription drugs.
Contact Number	(800) 250-8427

Vermont (continued)
Vscript and Vscript expanded

Eligibility	• Age 65 and older.
	• Income requirements must be met. Call for specifics.
	• Disabled and on Social Security.
	• Income eligibility higher with Vscript expanded.
How the Program Works	• Enroll.
	• Present the card at the pharmacy and pay a copay.
Cost to Join	None.
Copay	• $1 for prescriptions costing less than $29.99 and $2 for prescriptions costing more than $30.
	• 50% of retail cost for Vscript expanded.
Drugs Covered	Drugs for chronic diseases only.
Contact Number	(800) 250-8427

Vermont Division of Insurance   (800) 631-7788

WASHINGTON
A Washington Alliance to Reduce Prescription Drug Spending (AWARDS)

Eligibility	• Washington resident.
	• Age 55 and older.
	• No prescription drug coverage.
	• No income eligibility.
How the Program Works	• Submit application.
	• Pay the annual fee.
	• Receive a card.
	• Get the drug at discount prices set by Merck-Medco.
Cost to Join	Annual fee of $15 for single people or $25 for married couples.
Copay	None.
Drugs Covered	All drugs in Merck-Medco formulary.
Contact Number	(360) 923-2771

Washington State Insurance Department   (800) 562-6900

WEST VIRGINIA
Senior Prescription Assistance Network II (SPAN II)

Eligibility	• Age 65 and older.
	• No other prescription coverage.
	• Income requirements must be met. Call for specifics.
How the Program Works	• Apply and receive a card.
	• Present the card at a participating pharmacy.
	• Pay the discounted amount for the drug.
Cost to Join	None.
Copay	None.

West Virginia (continued)

Drugs Covered	All prescription drugs.
Contact Number	(877) 987-2622

West Virginia Insurance Commission   (800) 642-9004

Directory of Other State Health and Insurance Agencies

(*Note:* Phone numbers can change. If you call a phone number and it is not working, call information to get the new one.)

Alabama
Department of Public Health
(334) 206-5300

Department of Insurance
(334) 269-3550

Arizona
Health Care Containment System
(800) 654-8713 in State

Department of Insurance
(800) 325-2584

Arkansas
Department of Health
(501) 661-2000

Department of Insurance
(800) 852-5494

Colorado
Department of Health Care Policy and
  Financing
(303) 866-3513 (Metro Denver)
(800) 221-3943 (statewide)

Department of Insurance
(800) 930-3745

District of Columbia
Department of Health
(202) 442-9191

Department of Insurance and Security
  Regulation
(202) 727-8000

Georgia
Department of Community Health
Office of Communications
(404) 656-6359

Department of Insurance
(404) 656-2056

Hawaii
Department of Health
(808) 586-4400

Insurance Division
(808) 586-2790

Idaho
Department of Health and Welfare
(208) 334-5500

Department of Insurance
(208) 334-4398

Iowa
Department of Insurance
(515) 281-5705

Department of Public Health
(515) 281-4958

Kansas
Department of Health and Environment
(785) 296-1500

Department of Insurance
(800) 432-2484

Kentucky
Cabinet for Health Services
(502) 564-7042

Department of Insurance
(800) 595-6033

Louisiana
Department of Health and Hospitals
(225) 342-9500

Department of Insurance
(225) 342-7401

Mississippi
Department of Health
(601) 576-7400

Insurance Department
(800) 562-2957

Missouri
Department of Health
(573) 751-6400

Department of Insurance
(800) 726-7390

Montana
Department of Insurance
(406) 444-2040

Department of Public Health and
  Human Services
(406) 444-4540

Nebraska
Department of Insurance
(402) 471-2201

Health and Human Services System
(402) 471-2306

New Mexico
Department of Health
(505) 827-2613

Insurance Division
(505) 827-4601

North Carolina
Department of Health and Human
  Services
(800) 662-7030
  (North Carolina only)

Department of Insurance
(919) 733-6495

North Dakota
Department of Health
(701) 328-2372

Department of Insurance
(701) 328-2440

Ohio
Department of Health
(614) 466-5500

Department of Insurance
(800) 686-1526

Oklahoma
Department of Health
(405) 271-5600

Department of Insurance
(800) 522-0071

Oregon
Health Division
(503) 731-4000

Insurance Division
(503) 947-7980

South Dakota
Department of Health
(605) 773-3361

Division of Insurance
(605) 773-3563

Tennessee
Department of Commerce and
  Insurance
(800) 342-8385

Department of Health
(615) 741-3111

Texas
Department of Insurance
(800) 252-3439

Health and Human Services
  Commission
(512) 424-6500

Utah
Department of Health
(801) 538-6101

Department of Insurance
(801) 538-3800

Virginia
Bureau of Insurance
(800) 552-7945

Department of Health
(804) 786-0814

Wisconsin
Department of Health and Family
  Services
(608) 267-7371

Office of the Commissioner of
  Insurance
(800) 236-8517

Wyoming
Department of Health
(307) 777-7656

Department of Insurance
(800) 438-5768

Directory of Drug Companies' Patient Assistance Programs

All brand names are registered trademarks of the manufacturers.

Company	Name of Program	Phone Number
Abbott Laboratories	Uninsured Patient Program	(800) 222-6883
Agouron Pharmaceuticals	Viracept Assistance Program (VAP)	(888) 777-6637
Alza Pharmaceuticals	Indigent Patient Assistance Program	(800) 577-3788
Amgen	Safety Net® Program	(800) 272-9376
AstraZeneca	AstraZeneca LP Patient Assistance Program	(800) 355-6044
	Foscavir Assistance and Information on Reimbursement (F.A.I.R.)	(800) 488-3247
	Zeneca Pharmaceuticals Foundation Patient Assistance Program	(800) 424-3727
Bayer Corporation Pharmaceutical Division	Bayer Indigent Patient Program	(800) 988-9180
Biogen	Avonex Support Line	(800) 456-2255
Boehringer Ingelheim Pharmaceuticals	Partners in Health	(800) 556-8317
Bristol-Myers Squibb Company	Bristol-Myers Squibb Patient Assistance Program	(800) 332-2056
DuPont Pharmaceuticals Company	DuPont Pharmaceuticals Company Patient Assistance Program	(800) 474-2762

Company	Name of Program	Phone Number
Eisai	Aricept (donepezil HCl) Patient Assistance Program	(800) 226-2072
Elan Pharmaceuticals	Elan Pharmaceuticals Prescription Assistance Program	(800) 528-4362
Fujisawa Healthcare	Prograf Patient Assistant Program	(800) 4-PROGRAF
Genentech	Uninsured Patient Assistance Program	(800) 879-4747
Genetics Institute	The Benefix Reimbursement and Information Program	(888) 999-2349
	Neumega Access Program	(888) 638-6342
Genzyme Corporation	Ceredase/Cerezyme Access Program (CAP Program)	(800) 745-4447, ext. 7808
Gilead Sciences	Gilead Sciences Support Services	(800) 445-3235
Glaxo Wellcome	Glaxo Wellcome Patient Assistance Program	(800) 722-9294
Hoechst Marion Roussel (now Aventis Pharmaceuticals)	Patient Assistance Program	(800) 221-4025
	The Anzement Patient Assistance Program and the Anzement Reimbursement Program	(888) 259-2219
Janssen Pharmaceutica	Janssen Patient Assistance Program	(800) 544-2987
	Risperdal Patient Assistance Program and Risperdal Reimbursement Support Program	(800) 652-6227
Eli Lilly and Company	Lilly Cares	(800) 545- 6962
	Gemzar Patient Assistance Program	(888) 443-6927
The Liposome Company	Financial Assistance Program for Abelcet	(800) 335-5476
Merck and Company	Merck Patient Assistance Program	(800) 994-2111
	SUPPORT™ Reimbursement Support and Patient Assistance Services for Crixivan	(800) 850-3430
Novartis Pharmaceuticals	Novartis Patient Assistance Program	(800) 257-3273

Company	Name of Program	Phone Number
Ortho Biotech	Procritline	(800) 553-3851
Ortho Dermatological	Ortho Dermatological Patient Assistance Program	(800) 797-7737
Pasteur Mérieux Connaught	Indigent Patient Program	(800) 822-2463
Pfizer	Pfizer Prescription Assistance	(800) 646-4455
	Diflucan and Zithromax Patient Assistance Program	(800) 869-9979
	Sharing the Care	(800) 984-1500
	Aricept Assistance Program	(See Eisai)
	Lipitor Patient Assistance Program	(800) 646-4455
	(Participant in) Kentucky Health Care Access Program	(800) 633-8100
	(Participant in) Arkansas Health Care Access Program	(800) 950-8233
	(Participant in) Commun-I-Care	(800) 763-0059
Pharmacia	RxMAP Prescription Medication Assistance Program	(800) 242-7014
Procter and Gamble Pharmaceuticals	Customer Service	(800) 448-4878
Rhône-Poulenc Rorer (now Aventis Pharmaceuticals)	Rhône-Poulenc Rorer Patient Assistance Program	(610) 454-8110
Roche Laboratories	Roche Medical Needs Program	(800) 285-4484
	Roche Medical Needs Program (transplant reimbursement) for CellCept, Cytovene, and Cytovene-IV	(800) 772-5790
	Roche Medical Needs Program (HIV Therapy) for Fortase, Invirase, Cytovene, Cytovene-IV, and Hivid	(800) 282-7780
Roxane Laboratories	Patient Assistance Program	(800) 274-8651
Sanofi Pharmaceuticals	Needy Patient Program	(800) 446-6267
Schering Laboratories/ Key Pharmaceuticals	Commitment to Care	(800) 656-9485
Searle	Patients in Need®	(800) 542-2526

Company	Name of Program	Phone Number
Serono Laboratories	Connections for Growth	(617) 982-9000
	Serono Laboratories' Helping Hands Program	(617) 982-9000, ext. 5522
Sigma-Tau Pharmaceutical	NORD/Sigma-Tau Carnitor	(800) 999-NORD
	Drug Assistance (CDA) Program	(800) 999-NORD
	NORD/Sigma-Tau Matulane Patient Assistance Program	
GlaxoSmithKline	SKB Access to Care Program	(800) 546-0420
	Oncology Access to Care Program	(800) 699-3806
	Access to Care Paxil Certificate Program	(800) 729-4544
Solvay Pharmaceuticals	Patient Assistance Program	(800) 788-9277
3M Pharmaceuticals	Indigent Patient Assistance Program	(800) 328-0255
Wyeth-Ayerst Laboratories	Norplant Foundation	(703) 706-5933
	Rheumatoid Arthritis Assistance	(800) 282-7704
	Wyeth-Ayerst Laboratories Indigent Patient Program	(610) 688-4400

Directory of Some Internet Pharmacies

See chapter 5 for explanation of VIPPS certification.

Costco.com
www.costco.com
Costco.com is not listed as a VIPPS-certified site.

Cvs.com
www.cvs.com
Cvs.com is a VIPPS-certified site.

Drugstore.com
www.drugstore.com
Drugstore.com is a VIPPS-certified site.

Eckerd.com
www.eckerd.com
Eckerd.com is a VIPPS-certified site.

Familymeds.com
www.familymeds.com.
Familymeds.com is a VIPPS-certified site.

HorizonScripts.com
www.horizonscripts.com
Horizonscripts.com is not listed as a VIPPS-certified site.

PlanetRx.com
www.planetrx.com
PlanetRx.com is a VIPPS-certified site.

Pharmor.com
www.pharmor.com
Pharmor.com is not listed as a VIPPS-certified site.

Rx.com
www.rx.com
Rx.com is a VIPPS-certified site.

VitalRx.com
www.vitalrx.com
Vitalrx.com is a VIPPS-certified site.

Walgreens.com
www.walgreens.com
Walgreens.com is not listed as a VIPPS-certified site.

WebRx.com
www.webrx.com
Webrx.com is not listed as a VIPPS-certified site.

Keep in mind that web sites are constantly being redesigned and updated. The information provided here will most likely be modified as time goes by. Some sites might also cease operations while new sites are being added.

For more guidelines on what to look for when using a web site, call the FDA at (800) 463-6332, or log on to their web site at www.fda. gov/cder/drug/consumer/buyonline/guide.

For more information about certifying web sites and to check if a site has been VIPPS-certified, call the National Association of Boards of Pharmacy at (888) 481-9474, or visit their web site at www.nabp.net/vipps.

Directory of Some Discount Pharmacy Programs

AARP PHARMACY SERVICE

Membership Criteria	Must be a member of AARP
Cost of Membership	Comes with participating in AARP's insurance program; $15 a year if not participating in AARP's insurance program
Discount Promised	Lowest possible price offered by the pharmacy
Number of Pharmacies Participating	Nearly every pharmacy accepts the plan
Claim Forms	None
Deductibles	None
Other Benefits	AARP's total benefits package
Contact Number	(800) 532-5800
Web Address	www.aarphealthcare.com

AMERIPLAN

Membership Criteria	Open to everyone (not available in California)
Cost of Membership	$11.95 per month for individual and $19.95 per month for family
Discount Promised	Save up to 50% on most generics and up to 25% on most brand-name drugs
Number of Participating Pharmacies	Over 50,000 retail pharmacies nationwide
Claim Forms	None
Deductibles	None
Other Benefits	Chiropractic, dental, vision
Contact Number	(800) 797-2188
Web Address	www.ameriplanusa.com

AMERISAVE

Membership Criteria	Open to everyone
Cost of Membership	Ranges from $59 to $129 per year
Discount Promised	10 to 50% savings in neighborhood pharmacies, and more savings and a lowest-price guarantee with mail order purchases
Number of Participating Pharmacies	Over 45,000 chain and independent pharmacies
Claim Forms	None
Deductibles	None
Other Benefits	Discounts on vision, hearing aids, dental, chiropractic
Contact Number	(800) 800-7616
Web Address	www.amerisave.com

CATALYST SCRIPTS

Membership Criteria	Must be a member of a participating hospital senior membership program
Cost of Membership	Depends on the participating hospital
Discount Promised	10% to 50% on most drugs
Number of Participating Pharmacies	Over 48,000
Claim Forms	None
Deductibles	None
Other Benefits	Vision, dental, long-term-care planning, retirement seminars
Contact Number	(800) 814-0015
Web Address	www.catalystbenefits.com

DRUGCARD.COM

Membership Criteria	Open to all
Cost of Membership	$34.95 per year
Discount Promised	Up to 30%
Number of Participating Pharmacies	Over 48,000
Claim Forms	None
Deductibles	None
Other Benefits	Medical insurance, dental, doctor referrals
Contact Number	(800) 890-8170
Web Address	www.drugcard.com

MEMBERHEALTH

Membership Criteria	Open to all
Cost of Membership	$10 per year plus $5 per additional card for any family member
Discount Promised	20% to 70% on most brands
Number of Participating Pharmacies	Over 45,000
Claim Forms	None
Deductibles	None
Other Benefits	None
Contact Number	(888) 868-5854
Web Address	www.mhrx.com

NATIONAL ASSOCIATION OF MATURE AMERICANS

Membership Criteria	Open to all
Cost of Membership	$24.95 to $59.95 per year
Discount Promised	13% less than wholesale cost
Number of Participating Pharmacies	Over 40,000
Claim Forms	None
Deductibles	None
Other Benefits	Vision, medical equipment, hearing aids, magazines, flowers
Contact Number	(800) 409-0983
Web Address	www.namatx.com

PRESCRIPTION DISCOUNT PLUS

Membership Criteria	Open to all
Cost of Membership	$59.95 for individual and $89.95 for family per year
Discount Promised	Up to 50% on most prescriptions
Number of Participating Pharmacies	Over 40,000
Claim Forms	None
Deductibles	None
Other Benefits	None
Contact Number	(800) 454-7321
Web Address ·	www.prescriptiondiscount.com

PROCARE

Membership Criteria	Open to all
Cost for Membership	$15.95 per month plus a one-time $5 enrollment fee; additional $2.50 per card each for spouse or child
Discount Promised	10% to 40% on prescriptions
Number of Participating Pharmacies	Over 35,000
Claim Forms	None
Deductibles	None
Other Benefits	Discounts on doctor visits, pet coverage, lab test, home care, and nursing homes
Contact Number	(888) 750-4565
Web Address	www.procarecard.com

RX UNIVERSE

Membership Criteria	Open to all
Cost of Membership	$19.95 for individual and $34.95 for family per year
Discount Promised	5% to 80%
Number of Participating Pharmacies	Over 50,000
Claim Forms	None
Deductibles	None
Other Benefits	None
Contact Number	(800) 794-6490
Web Address	www.rxuniverse.com

SAVEWELL

Membership Criteria	Open to all
Cost of Membership	$52 per year
Discount Promised	Up to 50% off retail prices
Number of Participating Pharmacies	Over 50,000
Claim Forms	None
Deductibles	None
Other Benefits	Chiropractic, dental, vision
Contact Number	(877)-SAVEWELL
Web Address	www.savewell.com

SMARTCARD

Membership Criteria	Open to all
Cost of Membership	$49.95 per year
Discount Promised	Less than wholesale price
Number of Participating Pharmacies	Over 48,000
Claim Forms	None
Deductibles	None
Other Benefits	24-hour nurse assistance
Contact phone number	(800) 481-8405
Web Address	www.trsmartcard.com

YOURRXPLAN

Membership Criteria	Open to all
Cost of Membership	$25 single or $40 per family per year
Discount Promised	Less than wholesale price
Number of Participating Pharmacies	Over 40,000
Claim Forms	None
Deductibles	None
Other Benefits	Cash back on purchases of some medications
Contact phone number	(877) 733-6765
Web Address	www.yourrxplan.com

Index

asthma *(continued)*
  managing cost of, 131–37
  mechanisms of, 125–27
  medications for, 133–36
  physicians and, 132–33
  prevalence of, 125
  preventing and managing, 129–31
  resources, 138
  symptoms, 127
Asthma and Allergy Foundation of America,
  138

biofeedback, 160, 180
blood vessel damage, 186
bone loss. *See* osteoporosis
brand-name drugs, 33, 48–51
businesses, insurance and, 12, 14–15
buyer's clubs for HIV medications, 219
bypass surgery, 204

calcium, 225
cancer
  AIDS-related, 211
  causes of, 140–41
  defined, 140
  managing cost of, 144–46
  Medicare and, 145
  prevalence of, 139
  preventing, 142
  resources, 146
  screening and testing for, 144
  symptoms, 141
  treating, 145
  types of, 141–42
Cancer Information Service, 142
cardiovascular disease, 172, 173
caregiving, 106–107
Centers for Disease Control and Prevention
  (CDC), 208, 222
Centers for Medicare and Medicaid Services,
  81
CHAMPUS, 12
Child Health Insurance Program, 11, 136
chiropractic for arthritis, 123
chondroitin, 123
chronic diseases, 7, 35, 36–38, 40. *See also*
  specific diseases
clinical trials, 75, 106, 146, 218, 222
clinics, federally funded, 66, 170, 189, 215
COBRA, 15, 88–89, 90, 219
community hospitals, 69
compassionate use programs, 218–19
complementary medicine, 7. *See also*
  acupuncture; alternative therapies
conventional insurance plans, 13
conventional therapy, 7
copays, 34–35, 47, 63–64, 174

costs, healthcare
  direct, 1, 8
  hospitals, 5, 8, 71–76
  indirect, 1
  institutional care, 5, 7–8
  Medicaid and, 10
  Medicare and, 8–9
  nursing homes, 5, 8
  physician services, 63–67
  prescription drugs, 7, 9, 29–33
  primary prevention, 5–6, 17, 18, 22, 24–26
  pyramid of, 5–8
  secondary prevention, 6–7
  total, 5
Crystal Home Care, 171
CVS Pharmacies, 51

DASH diet, 196–97, 198
death and dying, dealing with, 93–94
deductibles, 47, 174
Department of Defense, 219
depression and anxiety
  anxiety defined, 149
  causes and course of, 147–48
  complementary and alternative therapies,
    159–61
  complications, 149, 151–52
  in diabetes, 178–79
  employment issues, 158–59
  family issues, 159
  general anxiety disorder, 151
  health professionals and, 153–55
  high-risk factors, 152
  hospitalization for, 158
  managing cost of, 152–58
  medications for, 155–58
  obsessive-compulsive disorder, 150
  panic disorder, 150
  phobias, 151
  post-traumatic stress disorder, 150
  prevalence of, 147, 148
  preventing, 152
  resources, 161
  St. John's wort for, 160–61
  suicide and, 149, 152, 158, 159
  symptoms, 148
  treatment of, 153
diabetes
  alternative remedies, 180
  complications, 171–75, 179–80
  diagnosing, 168–69
  employment issues, 177–78
  gestational, 165
  government programs for, 174
  hospitalization for, 173, 174
  managing cost of, 167–80
  mechanisms of, 162–63